Getting to Yum

ALSO BY KAREN LE BILLON
French Kids Eat Everything

Getting to Yum

The 7 Secrets of Raising Eager Eaters

KAREN LE BILLON

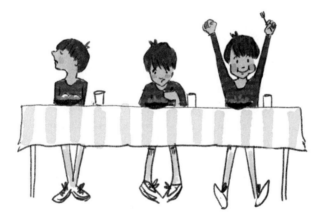

WM

WILLIAM MORROW

An Imprint of HarperCollinsPublishers

HarperCollins books may be purchased for educational, business, or sales promotional use. For information please e-mail the Special Markets Department at SPsales@harpercollins.com.

FIRST EDITION

Library of Congress Cataloging-in-Publication has been applied for.

ISBN 978-0-06-224870-1

14   15   16   17   18   [RRDH]   10   9   8   7   6   5   4   3   2   1

To Sophie and Claire, my best "taste testers"

Contents

GETTING TO YUM GAMES

Getting to Yum

Foreword

OBESITY RATES HAVE SKYROCKETED IN THE PAST SEVERAL DECADES, largely driven by unhealthful lifestyle behaviors in an increasingly automated "on the go" world. Aggressive food marketing has also fueled the childhood obesity epidemic by inducing children to crave high-calorie, low-nutrient foods and providing families with economic incentives to purchase them. Now more than ever, parents need effective strategies to help their children develop healthful eating habits for life.

As a pediatrician with expertise in pediatric obesity, one of the questions I am frequently asked is "How do we get children to eat what is good for them?" While this might seem like a simple question, the answer is incredibly complex. Karen Le Billon offered some thought-provoking ideas in her *New York Times* article "Why French Parents Are Superior (in One Way)." In it, Karen described how French parents effectively teach their children that "good-for-you foods" taste good, while American families often unwittingly do the opposite. In striking contrast to the limited repertoire of tastes preferred by many American children, the majority of French children learn to accept a large variety of tastes, flavors, and textures from an early age—and most of what they eat is healthy. As a matter of fact, North American children are three times more likely to be overweight than French children. Intrigued, I picked up a copy of Karen's first book, *French Kids Eat Everything,* and was transported to a small French town filled with wonderful flavors where Karen and her husband successfully converted their two children from picky eaters to foodie omnivores with the help of forward-thinking, government-backed nutrition policies and savvy parenting strategies.

In her long-awaited second book, *Getting to Yum*, Karen translates the current scientific evidence and her own experience transforming her children's eating behaviors in France into a treasure trove of valuable lessons to help parents everywhere to do the same. Her "Seven Secrets for Raising Eager Eaters" offer carefully researched, evidence-based yet highly practical advice to help parents tame finicky eaters. Karen provides a great explanation of how children develop tastes and how this impacts their willingness to accept new foods. She then offers insightful and practical strategies to get children to try new foods through taste-training experiments that teach children (and their parents) important but often-neglected food experience skills in a non-threatening and fun way. I was particularly impressed to see that Karen adopts the avant-garde concept of *parents themselves* marketing healthy foods to children; the latest research has shown this to be a much more effective approach than sneaking foods into children's diets.

As a medical educator and the mother of four children with very distinct personalities and taste preferences, I am always looking for evidence-based, adaptable, and user-friendly materials I can use at home and with my families at work. My sometimes-finicky children and I have had a lot of fun trying some of the taste experiments in this book (they recently discovered they like/are okay with grapefruit), and my kids have declared several of our "test" recipes positively yummy.

Getting to Yum is a must-read for parents who want to not only teach but also show their children that healthful foods can truly be "yummy." This book beckons families to embark on a taste discovery adventure and methodically shows them that food can be a great source of joy and exploration. I thoroughly enjoyed *Getting to Yum* with my family and hope that your family will, too. Welcome aboard!

Dr. Jennifer Cheng
Pediatrician and Clinical Director
One Step Ahead (Preventive Weight Management) Program
Harvard Medical School

Introduction

WHEN I FIRST MET JESSICA, HER 3-YEAR-OLD SON, LUCAS, WOULD not eat a single vegetable. Not one! Among Lucas's list of forbidden foods were meat (with the exception of hot dogs), "mushy" foods (even roasted potatoes), and "anything green." Jessica was at her wits' end. "The dinner table feels like a battleground. I leave feeling so stressed. My husband and I don't know what else to do," she told me.

A few months after adopting the taste-training method in this book, Lucas's eating habits dramatically improved. Previously off-limits foods were now among Lucas's favorites: green beans, oranges, grapefruit—even raw spinach. Best of all, Lucas's baby sister, who benefited from taste training right from the start, happily eats anything put in front of her. "As a result of taste training," Jessica explained, "we've adopted new routines that have changed our family's eating habits for the better."

What is taste training, and why is it useful for parents?

TASTE TRAINING IS A HANDS-ON, PRACTICAL APPROACH TO FOOD EDUCATION THAT uses games and fun activities to help children learn to like healthy foods. The underlying principle is that children can *learn* to eat well, just as they learn to read. The idea that taste can be taught is a hopeful, positive message. The goal is simple: children will enjoy eating healthy foods because they *want* to (not because they *have* to). Your children will develop positive eating routines (*how, where,* and *when* to eat) that foster balanced appetites and healthy attitudes to food. They'll be healthy, happy, savvy eaters.

Of course, many food cultures—the French, the Italians, the Japanese, to name a few—have been practicing their version of taste training for generations. It's only recently that scientists and educators have studied the effects of taste training, and explained how and why it works so well. Researchers have spent the past few decades doing hundreds of amazing (and sometimes downright funny) experiments on babies and children: feeding babies slightly acidic water (their "sour face" looks just like an adult's); asking toddlers to eat fake green "grasshopper" icing (they will, happily); or dyeing food blue to see if peer pressure works to encourage reluctant kids to eat "scary" things (it does).

The core message of the scientific research on taste training is simple and inspiring: kids can actually learn to like new tastes (even if they are cautious about them at first). And that's not all. Specific taste-training techniques improve children's eating habits, make them more willing to try new foods, and change their long-term eating habits for the better. Kids who have gone through taste training eat healthy foods more regularly and eagerly, even months after the taste training is over.In fact, scientific studies show that taste training works better than nutrition-focused education methods.

Our family's story: Curing picky eating

How do I know so much about kids and food? My best qualification is being a mom to two wonderful daughters who were both picky eaters (one of those "blessed obstacles" that was a source of enormous stress when I was a new mother). I'm also a university professor, so I love digging for answers to complex problems. These two parts of my identity collided when my husband and I moved to France with our two young daughters, who were then subsisting on a "beige food" diet (pasta, Cheerios, buttered toast, and crackers—you get the idea). Because taste training is widespread in French homes and schools, my daughters received a food education similar to what I describe in this book. Within a year, the two girls (then 5 and 2) were eating—and loving—a huge range of foods, including beet salad, creamed spinach, broccoli, and mussels. (No, I am not making this up!)

I was so inspired by the positive change in our family's eating habits—and convinced that we had learned life-changing lessons that could be of use to parents world-wide—that I wrote a book about our experience, *French Kids Eat Everything*, which has gone on to be published in a dozen countries and ten languages. Readers wrote to me with heartfelt stories about how the ideas in *French Kids* inspired them to feed their families better. Others requested more recipes, tips, and practical advice. "The memoir was a great read," wrote one mom, "but when are you coming out with *the* parenting book we're all looking for?" So I've spent the past two years exploring and integrating research from many different fields: education, medicine, neurobiology, nutrition, psychology, sociology, and even comparative anthropology. In *Getting to Yum*, I've distilled the results down into key lessons and strategies for parents. (And I let off steam in the kitchen by developing and testing the recipes on my own family!)

I've been blessed to share the journey of writing *Getting to Yum* with more than two dozen test families as well as more than 40 preschoolers at the Alphabet Academy in Connecticut. Their amazing stories and breakthroughs appear throughout this book and will, I hope, inspire you as much as they did me.

Could *my* family benefit from taste training?

HAVE YOU EVER FOUND YOURSELF THINKING ANY OF THESE THINGS:

- I know *what* my child should be eating, but I can't figure out *how* to get them to eat it.
- I want my child to eat better, but I don't want to use force, bribery, nagging, or begging.
- I often struggle to get my child to eat the recommended five servings of fruits and vegetables per day.
- My child reacts strongly or even refuses to eat when I serve new foods.
- I frequently make two or more meals at mealtime—one for the adults and one for each child.
- I sometimes substitute "kids' food" for healthier foods that my child rejects.
- Feeding my child is a source of stress.

If you responded "yes" to any of these statements, then this book is for you.

How does taste training work?

TASTE TRAINING HAS A SIMPLE GOAL: TO HELP YOU TEACH YOUR CHILD TO *enjoy* being a healthy eater. Because we often assume that kids' tastes are innate, teaching a child to eat might sound odd. How often have you heard a parent say, "My kid is such a picky eater"? We don't often think of eating as something that we *learn*; rather, we assume that eating is just something that we *do*. But kids *can* learn—and be taught—to eat well.

In order to achieve this goal, taste training involves three basic activities—fun games, simple recipes, and healthy eating routines—introduced in a strategic sequence: the "Seven Secrets" of healthy eating for kids. The underlying principle is that by improving *how, when,* and *why* you eat, you can improve *what* you eat.

Secret 1 explains how to *teach* your kids to enjoy tasting new foods. Secret 2 reveals how to use the power of food marketing to make healthy food more appealing for kids. Secret 3 helps you overhaul your family's eating routine through eliminating random snacking. Secret 4 introduces some mealtime magic: rituals and routines that make kids—and adults— eager to come to the table (and happy to stay there for a full meal). Secret 5 explains how to wean your kids off "kids' food" (if that's what they're used to eating). Most kids will feel more enthusiastic about this if they're helping in the kitchen—which is why Secret 6 is about child-led participation in cooking and family meal planning. And because parental emotions and attitudes are a key ingredient in your success, Secret 7 reveals techniques for keeping a Zen attitude despite the angst often associated with feeding our kids.

How do the games help?

Each of the Seven Secrets is associated with a set of fun games and experiments. Games are a fun, light-hearted, yet effective way to introduce your child to new ways of eating and to deepen their understanding of food. The taste-training games (some of which are actually basic science experiments) are based on principles of experiential education. The underlying idea is simple (and backed up by research): kids need to *experience* what they are learning, in a "hands-on" way, not simply be told what to do.Plus, games make learning to like new foods fun—for kids and adults alike.

Some of the games help children understand how eating relates to all five senses (touch, smell, sight, hearing, taste). As children become more comfortable with the physical sensations that different foods evoke, they become more confident eaters.For example, Game 9: The Sour Fruit Game on page 68 teaches children that a grapefruit tastes *sour*, but that this taste is *not unpleasant*. Many of my test families' children became grapefruit lovers after playing this game.

Other games are designed to solve (or prevent) common childhood eating issues, as shown in the list that follows. For example, children who have difficulty mixing foods of different textures may find Game 16: The Mixing Game to be helpful.

If your child has difficulty with this . . .	Try this . . .
Eating different foods mixed together	Game 16: The Mixing Game (page 118)
Accepting the texture of specific foods	Game 13: Terrific Textures (page 100)
Eating too quickly	Game 18: The Slow Food Experiment (page 131)
Disliking sour foods	Game 9: The Sour Fruit Game (page 68)
Accepting changes to their favorite dishes	Game 19: The Same Food Three Ways Experiment (page 132)
Being sensitive to strong tastes	Game 3: Tasty Taste Buds (page 35) Game 4: The Supertaster Game (page 37)
Refusing to eat healthy foods	Game 5: The Silly Name Game (page 52)
Preferring junk food to healthy food	Game 6: The Smell-Taste Experiment (page 53) Game 8: The Store-Brand versus Name-Brand Blind Taste Test (page 55) Game 14: The Color Confusion Experiment (page 104) Game 15: The Yogurt Game (page 105)
Sitting still at the table	Game 12: The Rose, Thorn, and Bud Game (page 86)
Eating salad	Game 17: Make-Your-Own Kids' Salad (page 120)

How do the recipes work with the taste-training approach?

THE RECIPES IN THIS BOOK ARE DESIGNED IN A SEQUENCE, WITH AGE-APPROPRIATE recipes for babies (approximately 9 to 18 months), toddlers (18 months to 4 years), pre-schoolers (4 to 6 years), and school-age children (6 years and older). The idea is simple:

just as you teach a child math in a series of small steps, so too do you teach a child to eat in a series of steps. You start by exposing babies to basic tastes (as you would teach them to count to 10). Then, you add textures, particularly at the toddler stage (as you would teach them to count even higher and introduce number sequences). Preschoolers then begin expanding their range of knowledge about food as they try new taste/texture combinations (addition and subtraction). Finally, they're able to eat like adults (advanced calculus—kidding!). The recipes are designed to follow this sequence, and progressively introduce more complex tastes and textures to your child's diet. Take red peppers, for example: the recipes include a Roasted Red Pepper and Tomato Soup (page 214) for babies, followed by Red Rocket Hummus (page 179) for toddlers, Pinwheel Pepper Wraps (page 216) for preschoolers, and Ratatouille (page 217) for older kids. The beauty of this approach is that each of these recipes is designed to be tasty for adults, too—even the purée, which is actually a simple soup.

The recipes are also designed to be deliberately adventurous. You might be surprised by some of the ingredients (such as sage or anchovies), but please put your doubts aside. You may find (as my test families often did) that your kids can enjoy these ingredients, even if they aren't usually considered typical kids' food.

Is taste training like sleep training?

EATING IS A BASIC BODILY FUNCTION, LIKE SLEEPING. BUT EATING WELL IS A COMPLEX skill that takes years to acquire. Taste training is best compared with reading. Learning to read well takes time and effort; it takes years before a child becomes a competent, confident reader. But this doesn't mean that reading is unpleasant. And neither is taste training. Curling up with a young child and reading them a book is one of the coziest things you could imagine. Remember how excited you were to rediscover your favorite kids' books with your child? Or what it was like when your child learned to walk or managed to bicycle on their own for the very first time? Now imagine you felt that way about teaching them about eating, about exploring the wonderful world of food together. What if you felt that way about introducing new foods—as something to be anticipated and celebrated?

Can *all* children learn to eat well?

YOUR BELIEF IN YOUR CHILD'S CAPACITY TO BECOME A COMPETENT EATER IS a key factor in their success. Some children will take longer (and some *much* longer) than others, but most children *can* learn to eat well. However, if your child seems to have particular difficulty eating, they may have an underlying medical issue (including allergies, autism spectrum disorder, or a sensory processing disorder) that is best dealt with in consultation with your health-care provider.

At what age can I start taste training?

TASTE TRAINING CAN BE STARTED AT ANY AGE. (IN FACT, SOME OF MY TEST families reported their biggest successes with formerly picky *parents*!) Although it is easier with younger children, it's never too late to start. If your children are older (as mine were when I started), don't worry: it may take a little longer, but kids are remarkably adaptable. For older kids, *Getting to Yum* can work as a "rehab" program, helping your children to wean themselves from processed foods and create new, positive eating habits. If you have a baby under the age of 2, your journey will be much easier. Taste training at this age is like preventive medicine. Your goal will be to nip picky eating in the bud and perhaps even prevent it from appearing altogether. Plus, you'll be able to take full advantage of the simple recipes at the back of this book. If you're starting at this age, you're lucky! You can create healthy eating routines right from the start.

Won't kids just grow out of picky eating on their own?

THE MAJORITY OF CHILDREN (AROUND THREE OUT OF FOUR IN MOST STUDIES) are selective about the foods they eat: rejecting new foods, preferring a small range of favorite foods, and even developing deep attachments to specific "fetish" foods (such as pasta). Pickiness, in other words, is normal for some children. But with simple taste-training techniques even the most hard-core picky eaters will diversify their diets.

At this point you may be congratulating yourself, saying, "My child isn't picky!" Good for you (and for them)—but don't celebrate too soon. Selective eating varies with age, in a fairly predictable pattern. It often appears during toddlerhood, but can also occur at other ages, for different reasons. About 4 out of 10 babies are eager eaters (particularly when they're hungry) who will enjoy or at least try new foods. Another 4 out of those 10 babies are strong-willed eaters who show strong food preferences right from the start. About 2 in 10 will be fussy eaters right from the start.

From about the age of 2 and up, some previously eager or strong-willed eaters will start to be selective. They might be fussy (refusing foods they've previously eaten and enjoyed, and often changing preferences from one day to the next) and/or picky (refusing to try new foods and making demands to eat familiar foods). Picky eating (termed "neophobia," or the fear of new foods) often emerges at around the age of 2 and usually peaks at about 4 or 5. Some research suggests that boys, on average, tend to be pickier than girls at this age.

By the time they start school, most children have a consistent sense of their likes and dislikes, and these preferences tend to remain stable over time. By the ages of 10 to 12, picky eating declines in most children, although food preferences change as children approach adolescence. If the family is experiencing power struggles over food, or an adolescent is experiencing other personal issues, pickiness may intensify. Pickiness may be related, for example, to concerns over personal health, body image, or eating disorders. Eventually, however, most children grow out of picky eating.

When this pattern of development was first explained to me, I was relieved. I realized that picky eating was a normal phase of development for many kids that arises from a combination of factors, including a child's innate eating type, family food habits and routines, and social pressures and experiences inside and outside the home. No more guilt! (Getting rid of guilt is one of the first steps in developing a healthy family eating routine.)

Most important, I also realized there was something I—and all parents—could do about picky eating. For most kids, picky eating is a phase, not a lifelong condition. Just as firm, responsive parenting can help kids grow out of the "no" phase, taste training can help your child grow out of picky eating.

What if my child resists? Won't it make picky eating worse?

IF YOU'RE WORRIED ABOUT RESISTANCE, START WITH THE GAMES LISTED IN each chapter. They're great for awakening your child's natural curiosity about food. They'll help you teach your child to like the taste of healthy foods and to adopt healthy eating habits throughout the day. The premise of this approach is that food is fun.

Yes, that's right. *Food is fun.* What does this mean? It means that you *can* enjoy meals with your children. You may not believe it right at this moment (and, believe me, when struggling with my young children's eating habits, I wouldn't have believed it either), but you and your child *can* have fun trying healthy new foods.

For really resistant kids, you might want to skip ahead to Secrets 6 and 7. Secret 6 explains how to replace pressure with kids' participation and introduces "child-led" learning strategies that are designed to get your child working with you rather than against you. Secret 7 has some suggestions for maintaining parental calm and detachment in stressful eating situations: the more relaxed (yet firm) you are when providing guidance, the more successful you are likely to be.

What about allergies?

TASTE TRAINING IS BASED ON THE BELIEF THAT WE DON'T NEED TO BE AFRAID of introducing a wide variety of foods and tastes to children of all ages (in fact, the younger the better). This approach is supported by recent medical advice that encourages parents not to delay the introduction of *any* foods—even those previously thought of as "allergenic"—to babies older than 6 months. In fact, doctors are now studying the possibility that delaying the introduction of allergenic foods—such as peanuts—may *increase* the chance of developing allergies. This idea (not yet scientifically proven) suggests that eating a wide variety of foods may actually protect against allergies. In summary, doctors recommend that a wide variety of foods be introduced early and eaten regularly. Taste training offers a method that enables you to put this advice into practice.

What taste training is not

TASTE TRAINING IS NOT A METHOD FOR PRODUCING "PERFECT" EATERS (there is no such thing). Nor does it assume that your child will eat everything. Children, just like adults, have taste preferences that should be respected.

Taste training is not about nutritional education. Extensive research shows that nutritional education is not very helpful for *changing* behavior or creating positive behaviors. In other words, getting your child to eat well has very little to do with nutrition. Don't get me wrong, nutrition is important—micronutrient deficiencies (particularly iron, zinc, and calcium) are still an issue for too many children, even in relatively wealthy societies—but research has shown time and again that using nutrition-based arguments is not the best way to convince your child to eat better.

Taste training is not a "blame and shame" approach to eating. Rather, it's a positive approach that treats food as a source of joy and exploration, like a shared adventure. It's about *how* we might inspire our children—and ourselves—to eat better, because it's something that they—and we—*enjoy* doing. So you won't hear me repeating the well-known information about the problems. Instead, we'll focus on solutions.

Finally, taste training is not about dieting or eating only "healthy" food (however that is defined). The recipes provided in the second part of the book focus on fruits and vegetables, which tend to be what children have a harder time learning to like. But I like to steer clear of labels (like "good" and "bad" foods). Rather, you'll teach your child that there are different approaches to foods: some they can eat regularly and some are occasional treats. My view is that there is nothing wrong with treats—in moderation. In fact, "moderation rather than deprivation" is a key *Getting to Yum* principle. Research shows that depriving children of certain foods makes them more likely to crave them. Equally, forcing children to eat "healthy" foods (or using treats as a bribe) makes it more probable that children will dislike those foods. Taste training takes a different approach: assuming that children can and will like all sorts of foods because they are inherently tasty. Broccoli . . . *yum!* That's why snack and dessert recipes are included, too.

How long will this take?

YOU MAY BE THINKING, SOUNDS GOOD, BUT HOW QUICKLY WILL I SEE A *change?* I won't kid you: it's not an instant process. Good eating doesn't happen overnight. If you're firm about the new approaches that you adopt, you will see changes in most toddlers within a week or two. School-age children will take longer. Adolescents might take up to a month or more. Be patient and gently persistent.

How much time per week will this take? If you play one game every day and introduce one new recipe a week, then you'll be spending 30 minutes a week on taste training—that's less than 5 minutes per day. Be warned, however: taste training grows on you. As my test families found out, once you start—and once your child surprises you with their breakthrough new food "likes"—you won't want to stop. (Food "breakthroughs" are mini triumphs that make your family food challenge a lot of fun.) Most test families found themselves doing more, not less, taste training over time.

Your family food journey is likely to be a bit of a rollercoaster ride. Your child will nibble on broccoli one day and balk at it the next. They'll whine at the table and forget their manners, then surprise you with their sweetness. Some family meals will be grumpy—this is where mindful eating can help. When applied to parents, I take it to mean "Take a deep breath, resist the temptation to yell or scold, and remember that this too shall pass." Remember that taste training, in the long run, will be worth it. You'll be spending less time in the kitchen because you'll be introducing the principle of "one family, one meal" to your household and eliminating short-order cooking. Your child will be less fussy at mealtimes and, in most cases, will have become an "easy eater." Ultimately, you'll be able to focus more on enjoying your child rather than being stressed about what they do (or don't) eat—and shouldn't that be the ultimate goal?

Let your family food adventure begin!

Love,
Karen

P.S. I've included lots of helpful extra information on **GettingToYum.com**, including recipes, menus, research sources, tips, and more. Check it out!

The Seven Secrets for Raising Eager Eaters

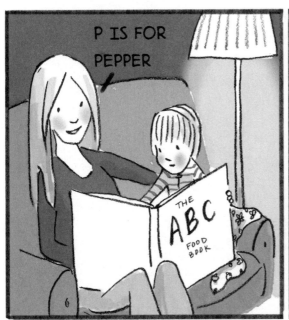

P IS FOR PEPPER

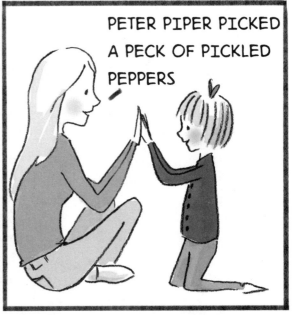

PETER PIPER PICKED A PECK OF PICKLED PEPPERS

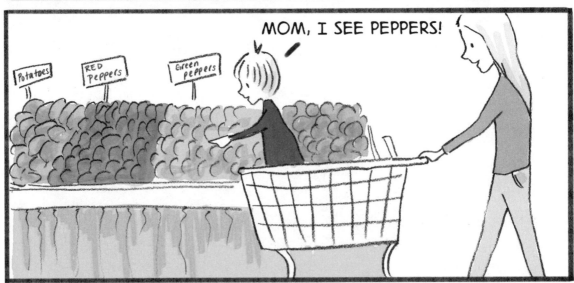

MOM, I SEE PEPPERS!

Kids Can *Learn* to Love Healthy Foods: Here's How to Teach Them

I MAGINE THAT ONE DAY YOU TRAVEL TO ANOTHER COUNTRY, SOMEWHERE far away, somewhere quite different. Soon after arriving, you meet a family with young children. Curious, the parents ask you to explain what children "back home" typically like to eat. What comes to mind? If you've been raised in North America, you probably thought of hot dogs, pizza, and soda. Or you might have thought of baby food: white rice cereal or maybe applesauce. Stereotypical kids' food.

Now imagine what happens when you ask that family what *their* kids eat. Depending on where you are, you'll get very different answers. In India, little kids eat curries (albeit milder versions than the adult variety); young children encounter herbs and spices like mint, turmeric, and cinnamon early on. Mexican toddlers begin eating hot sauce before they start first grade. In Korea, even young kids love sour kimchi (a pickled cabbage and vegetable dish), and a school lunch might include seaweed or bean sprout soup, pickled radish, or octopus stir-fry. In Japan, when not nibbling on *natto* (fermented soybeans), young children are served rice porridge topped with chopped tofu, fish (fresh or dried), or vegetables. In Italy, babies' cereals are mixed with *brodo* (a delicious vegetable broth seasoned with garlic and topped with Parmesan and olive oil). Jarred Italian baby food options include rabbit and even horsemeat. I've seen Italian mothers spoon-feeding café latté (presumably single-shot!) to their stroller-bound babies, both mom and tot cooing happily all the while. Seaweed and seal blubber (rich in vitamin C) are traditional first foods for Inuit babies, followed by whale meat and bush foods (such as caribou meat). In France, recommended first foods for babies include leek soup and endive. One of the top-selling French baby cookbooks includes vegetables such as artichoke, celery, and cauliflower for babies, and features dishes like sea bass with fennel ("Why not serve it for your child's first birthday meal?"). For the adventurous toddler, the same cookbook features "scallop tartare" (yes, raw seafood) topped with minced pickles, capers, and white pepper.

These examples might seem strange at first glance, but they're actually not. All over the world, parents introduce young children to the varied flavors of their particular food culture. That means introducing them to spicy foods, sour foods, salty foods, sweet foods—strong tastes of all kinds, even the ones that current North American culture would say kids "can't" like.

Your grandparents would probably have been perplexed by the idea of "kids' food"; when they were young, kids ate the same food as everyone else. This is, of course, partly practical: without refrigeration, and with seasonal (and often limited) food choices, people cooked what they had, and ate because they were hungry. Parents had no reason to believe that their kids wouldn't like the food that they ate. Industrial food culture has turned this relationship on its head. We now assume that kids prefer "kids' food," so that's (by and large) what we feed them.

But what if we took a more positive approach and assumed the opposite: that kids can actually *enjoy* eating a wide variety of foods? Why wouldn't we want children to enjoy the subtle flavor of, say, broccoli? If parents believe these vegetables are tasty and eat them themselves, their child will eventually learn to eat a healthy, diverse diet. And if a child is timid about a new vegetable and says "I hate it," a parent could (and should) help them figure out ways to like the new vegetable. As described in the experiment that follows, the starting point is your expectations of your child, which help set them up for success (or failure).

The Pygmalion Effect

HOW IMPORTANT ARE OUR BELIEFS ABOUT OUR CHILDREN'S CAPACITY TO learn? Very important, as Harvard researcher Robert Rosenthal found out. In 1965, Rosenthal (a psychologist) and Lenore Jacobsen (an elementary school principal) conducted an unorthodox experiment in a California public school. They told teachers that they had used a Harvard-designed test (the Harvard Test of Inflected Acquisition) to identify which students were about to go through an intellectual growth spurt. The teachers were excited, as the Harvard method was supposed to help them target and support kids' learning. But here's the thing about Rosenthal's experiment: it was based on a lie. The Test of Inflected Acquisition didn't exist. And the students identified as being about to "spurt" intellectually were chosen at random.

Rosenthal hoped to prove that teachers' expectations of students influenced how well students actually performed. He was proven right. When his team came back to the school several months later, the selected children had significantly improved their school performance. Even Rosenthal was surprised by how much the children had improved; he'd expected a small difference, but some children had gone from being C students to A students. He was also astounded by another result: the children had also gained in IQ, up to 40 points higher than the students who were not selected.

His conclusion? Teachers' expectations of how much children *could* learn powerfully influenced how much they *actually* learned. Rosenthal called this the "Pygmalion Effect," based on the famous play by George Bernard Shaw (and later the movie *My Fair Lady*) in which working-class Eliza Doolittle is taught by Professor Henry Higgins to lose her Cockney accent and adopt the manners of a lady, confounding the audience's beliefs about the natural inferiority of the "lower" classes.

Rosenthal's experiment had an enormous social impact because it proved that adults' expectations of children have an enormous influence on how children actually behave and learn—and the effect is most pronounced in young children. Perhaps most important, the experiment demonstrates the power of labels. If you label your son a picky eater, he will likely become one. If you tell your daughter there are some foods she doesn't like, she'll probably believe you. If you yourself believe that some foods (such as vegetables) are not tasty, your kids will probably feel the same way.

This notion of labels really hit home with my friend Kate, who only recently realized that her father didn't like broccoli yet dutifully ate it for 20 years. His devotion paid off: although he still doesn't like broccoli, it's Kate and her sister Lauren's favorite vegetable! The simple message: if you want your kids to eat something, eat it in front of them with obvious enjoyment. And tell them it's tasty.

The opposite is also true: if you act alarmed when your 3-year-old reaches for a piece of grapefruit (as one dad did when visiting our house for brunch) and say "Ooh, that's too acidic for you" in an alarmed voice (which is what he did), your toddler will probably recoil and decide she doesn't like it (which is exactly what his child did). Kids naturally feel wary of foods that their parents dislike. This behavior is, of course, a useful protective mechanism, but it can be taken too far. When your child encounters a new food, try simply encouraging them to try it—with curiosity and without judgment.

Kids are "emerging eaters"

INSTEAD OF LABELING YOUR CHILD A PICKY EATER, TRY THINKING OF THEM as a "learning" or "emerging" eater. Your child will believe that it's normal to learn to like new foods, and they'll naturally turn to you to help them to do so. If you avoid telling them (either directly or indirectly) that there are good- or bad-tasting foods, and rather describe food as having *interesting* tastes, they might surprise you with their interest in new foods.

Here's a simple example from our family. Last year we were at our local neighborhood block party in Vancouver, a city lucky enough to be home to a diverse set of cuisines. One of the treats on offer was a spicy snack: wasabi-flavored seaweed (wasabi—also known as Japanese horseradish—is a pale green paste with a hot mustard taste). Our neighbor offered me some, and then my 4-year-old daughter, Claire, asked for a piece. "Ooh, she'll find that too spicy, I think!" my neighbor replied as she angled the tray away from Claire. But Claire asked again, and I handed her half of my piece. As our neighbor backed up and waited for the (she thought) inevitable wail, I told Claire, "Try it—you'll like it. It's really tasty!" As Claire happily munched on her piece and asked for my other half, our perplexed neighbor tried one more time: "It's super-spicy, isn't it?" Claire nodded, while blithely savoring the snack and even asking for another piece.

This wasn't an isolated incident. Before the age of 5, Claire was also eating (and, more important, enjoying) Thai curries and tofu, sushi and spinach, broccoli and beets, Roquefort cheese, and more. This doesn't mean that she eats everything—she has a serious scrambled egg hang-up, for some reason—but she does eat most things. She and her older sister, Sophie (now 9), weren't born liking these foods, of course. They *learned* to enjoy eating them. In fact, young kids are open to eating a much broader range of foods than we think.

There's a comb in my milk . . . *yum!*

INTRIGUED BY YOUNG CHILDREN'S ATTITUDES TOWARD FOOD, PAUL ROZIN (a psychologist at the University of Pennsylvania) decided to study how humans develop feelings of disgust. His experiments were simple. In one case, children listened to a story in which a contaminant (a grasshopper, a leaf, and even "doggie doo") falls into a glass of milk. After each sentence, children were asked how much they would like to drink the milk, rating their responses with a smiley face chart. Another experiment asked children to consume foods that seemed to be contaminated; for example, the experimenter pretended to comb their hair, then dipped the comb in a glass of juice, removed it, and asked the child to drink the juice. Over the years, the experimenters tried many different strategies, including my favorite: asking toddlers to eat shortbread sprinkled with "grasshopper powder" (flour, sugar, green food coloring). The adults who participated in the experiment were exposed to additional scenarios, which included stirring soup with a never-used comb or flyswatter.

How did the kids and adults react to Rozin's experiments? Older kids wouldn't even dream of accepting the drink or soup until the glass was washed—and even then, half of them still refused. The adults were the most resistant: many not only refused to taste, but suggested the now-contaminated glass or bowl should simply be thrown out. However, the youngest children (3-year-olds) were happy to sip their milk, slurp their juice, and chomp their grasshopper powder–topped cookies. They didn't appear to distinguish between foods that were dangerous, disgusting, or simply inappropriate.

As Rozin summed it up: "Young children seem to believe that things that are bad for them will taste bad. And things that are good for them will taste good." So how does a child learn that broccoli is good *and* tastes good, too? Not on their own, Rozin's research suggests. Rather, children learn food *dislikes* from the adults and other kids around them. And as every parent knows, food preferences are hard to change once they're established.

Supertasters

KIDS ARE NOT A BLANK SLATE, HOWEVER. RECENT DISCOVERIES HAVE SHOWN that taste sensitivity is, to some extent, genetic. University of Florida researcher Linda Bartoshuk studies the genetic variations in taste perception and categorizes people three ways: supertasters, average tasters, and non-tasters.

For supertasters, about 25 percent of the American population, bitter foods taste much more bitter and sweeter foods much more sweet. "Average tasters" make up 50 percent of the population. The remaining 25 percent are the "non-tasters," who are much less sensitive to any taste sensation. As Bartoshuk explains, "Supertasters live in a 'neon' world of taste, while non-tasters are in a 'pastel' world."I think I have one child on each extreme of the spectrum: my older daughter will gasp in pain and immediately spit out any raw garlic that accidentally finds its way into her food. My younger daughter will, on the other hand, chew on it thoughtfully, without much obvious discomfort. This doesn't mean that my older daughter doesn't enjoy strong flavors (she loves Thai curry, for example), but it does take her a little longer to learn to like them.

Why are kids so different from one another? Part of the reason may be physiological: they may have a different density of fungiform papillae (taste buds). Each taste bud is associated with a bundle of nerves that sends pain signals to the brain. More taste buds translate to stronger pain sensation, and more sensitive taste perception in general. (Interestingly, women are more likely to be supertasters because they tend to have more taste buds than men.)

The important thing to remember is that children have (on average) more taste buds than adults. In other words, most children will have a more sensitive sense of taste than most adults. This is why lots of practice—through repeated tasting of new foods—is so important: *most* kids are likely to take longer than the average adult to get used to the new tastes of foods. Patient, gentle persistence is key to taste training.

Don't be worried about "funny faces"

WHEN SERVING NEW FOODS TO YOUR CHILDREN, BE AWARE THAT THEIR facial expressions may be misleading. Scientists have found that children's facial expressions are a good indicator of food likes, but not of food dislikes. No one is sure why kids make such faces, but their expression may be a hangover from the "gusto-facial reflex" that newborn babies display when given acidic or bitter tastes. Even though kids have a cautious look on their face, or even wrinkle up their noses, that doesn't mean they dislike the new food. Rely on what children say rather than how they look.

THE GUSTO-FACIAL REFLEX

What happens if you give an infant a sip of a sweet liquid? And then a sour liquid? It turns out that all infants show the same reactions: happy-looking faces for sweet tastes, and grimaces for sour (and bitter and salty) tastes. These reactions are so universal, and so easily discernible, that when researchers took photos of the babies' faces and showed them to uninformed adults, the adults were easily able to tell what the babies had tasted. The gusto-facial reflex appears in the first day of life in children all over the world. Scientists thus term it an innate (observed at birth) reflex, rather than an acquired (or learned) reflex. It likely evolved due to its protective qualities (breast milk is sweet, and many toxins and poisons taste bitter). Children gradually learn to like a variety of tastes, but their "funny food faces" (which could to some extent be inadvertent) may persist until adolescence.

Practice, practice, practice

WHEN WAS THE LAST TIME YOU LEARNED TO LIKE A NEW FOOD? FOR MOST OF us, it was a while ago. Just like kids, we get stuck in food habits. We've forgotten that we actually had to learn to like the foods we now enjoy (it took me years to enjoy the taste of coffee, for example). The good news is that kids (and adults, too) can learn to like new foods through repeated exposure: basically, practice makes perfect.

Of course, you can overdo practicing. This is particularly the case for younger children (up until about the age of 7 or 8), for whom trying new foods is sometimes a big challenge. Introducing too many new foods to younger kids all at once might backfire, as they need a slower pace. It's about finding a balance: some variety and new foods, but not too much. Once per day may work for many kids, but once per week might be better for others. You know your child best.

Just a little regular practice can bring results very quickly; having your child spend only 5 minutes per day trying new foods and practicing their habits quickly adds up. This is important because studies show that, on average, children need to taste a new food anywhere up to 12 times before they will happily eat it. For example, 4-year-old Rena (one of my test family kids) wasn't so sure about cauliflower the first two times it was served. But the third time her mom Babette served the Cauliflower Gratin (page 196), both Rena and her little sister ate it without complaint (and even asked for more).

Jon (from another test family) had a similar experience with his 13-year-old son, Michael, a confirmed picky eater. Described by his dad as "a kid who had probably never tried a green bean," Michael tried (with some reluctance) Green Beans Amandine (page 202). The first time, he didn't finish his serving or express interest in having any more. The next week, however, Michael surprised his entire family by asking, "Why can't we have green beans more often?" Jon wrote to me afterward:

My wife and I were speechless. Now my son is asking for green beans! Remarkable. Illustrates how we let our misconceived assumptions about what children like and don't like get in the way of actually helping our kids to learn to like food.

— JON

As both Michael and Rena's examples show, repeated *low-pressure* exposure to new food is critical to successful taste training. That's why I recommend that your family adopt this simple—but extremely effective—Family Food Rule:

You don't have to like it, but you do have to taste it.

Some readers will recognize this as one of the Food Rules I described in *French Kids Eat Everything,* written after our family spent a year in France. There, we saw the impressive (seemingly magical) results of asking children to taste everything prepared for them, even if they don't eat it. The more familiar something is, the more children tend to like it. Your goal is to build that familiarity through regular repetition. Note: looking at the food isn't enough—children have to taste it (remember, it may take up to a dozen "tastes" before your child will eat a new food). Cautious kids will benefit from other types of exposure first: seeing, touching, and talking about the new food.

Children quickly learn this rule, and sometimes even encourage each other to follow it, as did Rena (one of my test family kids). Only a few days into the taste-testing process, Rena started asking her parents what she would be eating for dinner. Meals became something to look forward to, to be curious about. Rena was proud of being the "big kid," chanting "you don't have to like it, you just have to try it" to encourage her little sister, Rachel (2½), to follow suit. Rachel even surprised her parents by being the more eager eater, particularly when brightly colored foods were served.

Even young children can encourage one another to taste test new foods, as Alexandra, a reader, wrote to me:

> *I made a version of Ratatouille today with vegetables we grew in our garden. With spoon in hand, my 2½-year-old son sat at the lunch table staring at his bowl and not touching a bite. Then, between mouthfuls, my 4-year-old daughter simply said, "You don't have to like it, but you have to try it." And try it he did . . . until his whole bowl was empty and he asked for more.*
>
> —ALEXANDRA

Banish the bland

LEARNING TO LIKE NEW THINGS IS EVEN MORE COMPLICATED IF YOUR CHILD prefers a fairly bland diet. The problem with the bland food approach is that it teaches kids to avoid strong tastes—which is what characterizes most healthy food. When they grow older, we worry that they don't eat their recommended 2½ cups of vegetables and fruits per day. And we *should* worry: child obesity rates are rapidly rising around the world, affecting our children's mental and physical health, their school performance, even their IQ.

Dr. Jatinder Bhatia, a pediatrician and member of the American Academy of Pediatrics Committee on Nutrition, recommends feeding mild curries to babies.Indian parents feed curry to their babies from a very early age. The result is that they develop their baby's love of curry taste *before* they arrive at the "no" stage at around age 2. The same reasoning applies to all sorts of cultures, including Japan, where parents feed fish (*shirasu*) to infants.

The lesson here is simple: if you focus on developing a baby's palate early on, they'll be less likely to be extremely picky later in life. This is one reason parents from other cultures are often mystified upon learning that North Americans serve mostly bland food to their babies. When I explained the approach recommended in my American baby books to my French friend Laurence, she asked, puzzled, "Are you training them to *dislike* most foods?"

This doesn't mean you should serve a blazingly hot curry to your 3-year-old tonight. It's a gradual process. Being good at something doesn't happen overnight. If you've ever taught a child to ride a bicycle, swim, or play the piano, you know that it takes time. *Lots* of time. Patient persistence is a parent's best friend. You may be surprised, like Françoise:

> *I never had the confidence to push new dishes and vegetables. I backed down too fast. Now I am more confident to keep trying things they've said they didn't like for years. I've been surprised by what my kids like and don't like, and have discovered many things about each child's preferences (I thought I knew them!). My 3-year-old was, I thought, my easiest eater, but then I realized that she liked healthy things but not necessarily new things—totally different. I'm also surprised that they liked the most adventurous tastes (apple curry soup) but not the sweet things (berry yogurt). We ordered lamb at a restaurant the other day, and they were fighting over it! So their taste buds have definitely developed.*
>
> —FRANÇOISE

Do your kids (and yourself) a "friendly flavor" favor

MANY KIDS DON'T LIKE THE TASTE OF VEGETABLES ON THE FIRST TRY. Nature seems to have unfairly stacked the deck. The tastes that our kids seem to love are exactly the same as the ones we can't resist as adults: sugar above all, but also salt and fat. In fact, as the processed food industry has discovered, the right combination of sugar, salt, and fat can even result in addiction-like symptoms in both kids and adults.

The power of innate taste preferences is evident right from birth: newborns love sugar.A drop of a sweet taste on an infant's tongue will result in a smile and the relaxation of baby's muscles—so much so that doctors call this the "analgesic" (pain-reducing) effect of sugar, and have actually tested the use of sugar solutions as a means of reducing infant pain during medical procedures. (I don't think I would have signed up my girls for this experiment, but I'm glad some brave parents did.) Conversely, a drop of a sour taste will result in a reflex response that any parent will recognize: that dreaded pursing of lips and furrowing of brow that means "I don't like it!"

The preference for sweet isn't limited to North American food culture. Children around the world tend to prefer sweet, salty, and fatty flavors, and to be less fond of the sour, bitter, alkaline flavors that characterize vegetables. (Scientists don't know why this is the case but believe that it may be due to an innate aversion to potential toxins and poisons, which tend to be sour and bitter.) It's no surprise that children like those same vegetables much more if they are flavored with a little fat (a dollop of butter, a drizzle of olive oil) or naturally sweet foods (leek purée mixed with a little pear, for example).

As you're conducting taste experiments at home, keep in mind that some children may benefit from the "friendly flavor" tactic. Simply put: if you use flavors your child already enjoys, they will be more willing to try (and more likely to enjoy) new foods. Scientists call this effect "flavor conditioning," and have done many experiments on why and how it works.In one experiment, researchers added white sugar to grapefruit and found that children increased their liking for not just grapefruit but all sour foods as a result.Interestingly, serving flavorful preparations of fruits and vegetables to kids increased their subsequent liking for the plain versions of the vegetables; kids will "graduate" from grapefruit with sugar to plain grapefruit (as mine have done).

Many parents use "flavor conditioning" already (think ketchup, at least in North America). There are lots of flavors to try: my kids love "green ketchup" (*Pistou*, page 305), a yummy veggie pesto sauce. Classic Vinaigrette (page 303) is a great dip for all sorts of vegetables (or use a salad dressing that your children like). Or keep it simple: butter or olive oil, with a pinch of salt, works wonders with most vegetables. Whatever condiments you choose (hummus, sweet-and-sour sauce, yogurt dip, or even ketchup) are fine; just be sure to expose your child to more than one "friendly flavor." Resist the temptation to coat everything in tomato ketchup! You want to program your child to prefer the taste of real food and to expect variety—not to get stuck liking just a few things. The more you can vary these flavors, the better.

Using the friendly flavor approach is a great way to gradually taste train your kids: you can use familiar flavors as building blocks to introduce more complex dishes to your child's repertoire. For example, our friend Laurence, who lives in the south of France, started off serving simple zucchini purée to her baby Antoine, then added parsley and tomatoes a few months later. By the time baby Antoine was a 1½ years old, eggplant and peppers had been added, the texture had gone from smooth to lumpy, and Antoine was eating something that closely resembled the classic French stew ratatouille (recipe page 217).

How to teach a child to learn to like new foods

What would you do if a child was timid on the first day at a new school and said "I hate school"? You'd help them figure out ways to like school. You'd gently persist. Learning to like new foods—often one at a time—is similar.

How do you introduce new foods in a way that respects children's individual sensitivities? And how do you do this without force (which almost inevitably backfires)? One of the best ways is the taste test approach, in which you ask a child to taste a small amount but don't require them to eat it. When a child says "I don't like that food," they often mean "I don't know it." Being exposed to a new food in multiple ways helps children to tame their fears.

> When we started taste testing and thinking about food like a mini-experiment, I began asking my kids questions when they didn't like a particular recipe. What don't you like: the texture, the smell, the appearance, or the other ingredients? This encouraged my kids to explore the depth of food and food combinations. Through this process, we discovered Kelly actually did like soup, but didn't enjoy the texture of celery, which was a huge breakthrough for her (the one person who didn't like soup in our soup-o-phile home). It was also through this process that I confirmed that my daughters

found dressing to be too spicy, and lettuce too hard to get on a fork. That led me to rework the way I prepare salad, which they now love!

—LORI

A word of warning: avoid trying new foods if your child is feeling ill or if you're about to go on a long car ride and you know your child has a tendency to get carsick. Psychologists have found that humans are hard-wired to develop aversions to food they associate with illness: if you feed a person a new food and then make them feel ill shortly after, they'll develop an aversion for the odor and flavor of that food—even if it wasn't the cause of their illness. But don't worry: if your child does develop a food aversion in this way, it probably won't last forever.

Ready, set . . . taste!

SO HOW DO YOU PUT THE IDEAS IN THIS CHAPTER INTO ACTION? FIRST, YOU can teach your child how to learn to like new foods using the step-by-step taste-testing method that follows. Once they've got used to taste testing, you can introduce new foods using the easy-to-make recipes in the second part of this book. You can also try following the family taste-testing plan on page 32. After that, you can use the four games starting on the same page to introduce your child to some basic ideas about flavors and taste buds that will encourage them to broaden their palates. (Feel free to change the order of any of these steps to suit your family.)

Taste Testing: A Step-by-Step Approach

1. **Pick a new food similar to something your child already likes.** If they like cucumbers, try thin slices of green pepper. If they like carrots, try red peppers. If they like one kind of bread, try a different kind of bread.
2. **Introduce it before you serve it.** Sounds silly, but this step is important because children are often wary of foods they don't recognize. For example, show your child a red pepper (the sweet, not spicy kind!). Go shopping with them and let them choose one to take home. Better yet, find one growing in a garden. Let them touch it and smell it. Cut it open and let them look at the intense color. Next, try a variety of ways to introduce red peppers to your family. Children may appreci-

ate helping with cooking and serving "their" chosen vegetable. This will also help them make the connection between foods in different forms—that raw tomato they're wary about tasting is the main ingredient in the pizza sauce they love. Introducing children to raw vegetables often helps them overcome their wariness of eating vegetables in cooked form.

3. **Serve a small amount, prepared as plainly as possible, but still packed with flavor.** Use a little tasting bowl or ramekin, or serve a taste on a small spoon. A little bit of carrot soup on a spoon looks a lot less intimidating than a huge bowl of soup on the table. For cautious kids, you can try putting a small dollop or dab of the new food on one of their favorite crackers (or simply bread, if they prefer that). Some children will be reassured if they're allowed to dab the food on the cracker themselves.

4. **Taste it yourself—and enjoy it!** Research shows that kids are more likely to be willing to try (and actually eat) a food if parents or peers try it first— and visibly enjoy it. (Don't fake it—they'll have you figured out in a flash.)

5. **Don't ask them to eat it; simply ask them to taste it.** The key is not to create stress around accepting or rejecting new foods. Simply ask the child to taste and get acquainted with the dish. Removing the pressure to eat (by asking them to just taste) means that they aren't resisting—they're just experimenting, in a low-pressure and encouraging environment. Try telling them, "Don't let the eyes do the work of the tongue." Kids judge foods primarily by appearance (color and texture). This means they're more likely to be wary of new things. If you sprinkle chopped fresh parsley on their favorite pasta, their suspicions will be raised, even if it tastes pretty much the same. Encourage them to move beyond first impressions and actually taste things rather than pre-judge them. You might also want to tell reluctant children that they're allowed to spit the food out (as politely as possible) or to simply test it with their tongue. In other words, they don't have to swallow the food that they're taste testing. Most important, try not to react negatively if your child decides not to eat the new food. A cheerful, firm comment ("You'll like it more the next time") sends the right message.

6. **Ask your child to talk about it.** Whatever you do, don't ask your child if they like the new food—you'll be setting yourself up for a "No!" Rather,

ask them to describe the food in positive (or at least neutral) terms. If kids get used to saying "yuck" about anything unfamiliar, they'll risk getting stuck in a food-refusal rut. Describing the foods will help make the food more familiar. Ask your child to tell you what they think about the actual taste of the food, commenting on the flavors and textures they're encountering. Think of fun words you can teach your child to describe the different attributes of the food they are tasting: temperature (icy, lukewarm, steaming, scalding), taste (bitter, acidic, honeyed, savory, spicy, sweet-and-sour, tangy, zesty), texture (creamy, crunchy, crispy, crumbly, dry, fatty, fizzy, flaky, silky, tender, tough). Have fun thinking of new words or even inventing them—my younger daughter, Claire, likes to describe desserts she loves as "plummy." By giving your child the language to describe their food, you'll find out what they like (as well as what they don't like) and be able to adjust your cooking accordingly. So if the red pepper is "too crunchy" the first time you try it, you might try roasting it for the next taste experiment.

7. **Rotate the new food into your family meals regularly.** How often will depend on your child; some will be open to new foods several times a week, whereas others may find that a little overwhelming at first. Older children will be able to handle more variety (for example, raw red pepper in a salad one day, roasted red peppers another day), but younger children may prefer less variety. You know your child best.

8. **Keep trying (the "Delicious Dozen" rule).** Don't give up if the food is rejected once, or twice, or even more often than that. Be persistent (but not insistent). The new food in question should reappear on your family menu regularly at least until your child learns to like it. If they don't like it, don't react. Instead, tell them "You're still learning to like it" or "You'll like that when you're a bit more grown-up" or "You just haven't tasted it enough times yet." It's important that older children, in particular, give new foods a chance. Remind them that children need to taste (some) new foods up to a dozen times before they become familiar enough to be eaten—our family calls this the "Delicious Dozen" rule. Kids love to count (particularly younger kids). Even older ones like the challenge of remembering how many times they've tasted something.

Of course, you can adapt taste testing in any way that works for your family. One of my test family moms, Stacy, tried introducing new foods as a snack instead of as a meal. Stacy found that this made taste testing more casual. With less pressure, she had better results with her 6- and 4-year-old boys. One day, for example, Stacy handed her kids a raw cranberry at snack-time, without any pressure to try it. They each took a bite! They tasted the cranberries again at afternoon snack the next day, after they had been dusted with sugar. That evening, Stacy added some dried cranberries to their dinner salad and they ate them all up.

Martha had a similar success. After months of trying—without success—to get 3-year-old Tobias to eat potatoes, she decided to try a taste-testing approach. She bought very small new potatoes, which are a little sweeter than the large potatoes she usually bought. She served them whole, as usual. "They look cute," said Tobias. Previously, Martha had served the potatoes already peeled and mashed them for Tobias on his plate. But this time, Tobias and Martha peeled them together at the table, and Tobias mashed them himself on his plate. Result? "Oh, Mommy, I love them!"

A family food challenge: Four weeks, four new foods

AFTER YOUR CHILD HAS LEARNED THE BASICS OF TASTE TESTING, YOU CAN try introducing new foods regularly. The recipes that start on page 175 are designed to make this easy for children of all ages. For example, kids of any age will enjoy the Amazing Avocado Smoothie (page 251), which also works well for babies. As your baby grows, the recipes become more complex: you can serve the Avocado Smoothie to your baby, Beginner's Guacamole (page 252) to your toddler, and then Avocado Salsa Salad (page 254) to older children and adults. For older children who are cautious eaters, you can go back to the start, introducing these recipes in sequence: start with the smoothie; when they like that, follow up with the guacamole; and eventually, when they're ready, introduce the Avocado Salsa Salad—not forgetting the Awesome Avocado Ice Pops (page 254)! All of the recipes are designed to be used in a similar way: they can "grow" along with your child or be used in sequence to introduce older children to new foods and tastes.

How quickly should you try introducing each new food? I recommend creating a taste-testing plan, trying one new vegetable at a time. Most of my test families found that one vegetable per week was a good pace. Some families (with younger or more cautious kids) tried the same recipe multiple times. Other families (with older or more adventurous kids) tried different recipes using the same vegetable. The recipes are organized by vegetable, and there are four options per veggie—lots to choose from!

Your family taste-testing plan

IT MIGHT SEEM SILLY TO HAVE A FORMAL TASTE-TESTING PLAN, BUT MANY children enjoy it. One of my taste-testing dads, Jon, printed the plan out and put it on a clipboard with a pen. His teenage children were impressed and took the exercise more seriously. Roberta posted her worksheet on the fridge, and her three boys (3, 5, and 7) loved writing down (with some help) their thoughts about the recipes.

You can download a printable version of this worksheet at **GettingToYum.com**.

Taste-Testing Worksheet

Vegetable	Taste Test #1	Taste Test #2	Taste Test #3	Taste Test #4
Broccoli	Recipe: Our thoughts:	Recipe: Our thoughts:	Recipe: Our thoughts:	Recipe: Our thoughts:
Carrots	Recipe: Our thoughts:	Recipe: Our thoughts:	Recipe: Our thoughts:	Recipe: Our thoughts:
Cauliflower	Recipe: Our thoughts:	Recipe: Our thoughts:	Recipe: Our thoughts:	Recipe: Our thoughts:
Green beans	Recipe: Our thoughts:	Recipe: Our thoughts:	Recipe: Our thoughts:	Recipe: Our thoughts:

Four fun games

THESE GAMES INTRODUCE BASIC IDEAS ABOUT TASTE BUDS IN ORDER TO GIVE children a deeper understanding of their sense of taste. If your child is keen, you can try all four games. Otherwise, I recommend picking the age-appropriate game that you think will interest your child the most.

Game 1: The Five Senses (Ages 4 and Up)

MAIN MESSAGE:

This game is designed to help your child get excited about learning about food through investigating the five senses: sight, touch, hearing, smell, and taste. This will allow your child to better understand their reactions to foods (both ones they like and ones they don't like). Ideally, play this at snack-time (when they are hungry, but not too hungry).

WHAT YOU'LL NEED:

One of your child's preferred foods (ideally a fruit or vegetable)

WHAT TO DO:

Pick a food you know your child likes to eat—a favorite fruit or vegetable is ideal—and wash and prepare it together. For example, if you were to pick an apple, you might core and slice it. Sit down with your child and let them know you're going to play a snack-time game. Let them see that you're excited and interested in their reaction. Then ask your child this series of questions. Be positive and encouraging no matter how they answer, and feel free to change up the dialogue to fit your needs.

Which foods do you like to eat?
Show them the food.
Which part of your body do you use to see?
Show them the food again, then ask: What do you see?
Which part of your body do you use to smell?
Ask them to smell the food, then ask: What do you smell?
Which part of your body do you use to touch?
Let them touch the food, then ask: What does it feel like?
Encourage them to use words by asking follow-up questions about texture. For example: Is it smooth or bumpy? Is it hot or cold? Is it sticky?
Ask them to "test" the food by tasting it, then ask: What does it taste like?
Encourage them to use words like "sweet," "salty," "sour," "crunchy," and so on.
What noise do you hear when eating it?
Once the child is done, ask: How does your mouth feel? Do you taste the food?

Repeat the game with other foods your child likes until they're comfortable with it. Then repeat this game with a new food your child has recently learned to like or with a new food that you believe they are quite likely to enjoy. Don't ask them to eat the food, but just to test it (which could mean simply licking it or putting it in their mouth to chew without necessarily swallowing). It's best if you make your initial taste-testing choices simple: a piece of dried or fresh fruit, for example. Gradually, repeat the game with more and more complex or "difficult" foods. Remember, don't judge their reactions. Simply ask them to describe the food. Be as curious as you hope they will learn to be.

Chat about it. Many test families found that this game worked wonders with their younger children. The key is to ask kids to talk about the experience. As children do this, they learn to observe their reactions rather than simply react to anything new in a negative, knee-jerk way. As you encourage your child's natural curiosity, they'll grow more confident about taste testing. Respect their opinions. If they don't like something, that's fine. Ask them to explain why (to the limits of their ability, of course). Over time, this game will help your children become more open to trying new foods. Above all, make it fun.

Game 2: The Five Flavors (Ages 4 and Up)
MAIN MESSAGE:
This game introduces your child to the five different categories of flavors: sweet, salty, sour, bitter, and umami (savory)—which roughly translates from Japanese as "deliciously yummy." Umami is best described as a round, pleasant, savory or meaty or broth-like taste; it is found naturally in some fish and shellfish, certain vegetables (such as mushrooms, ripe tomatoes, spinach, and *kombu* seaweed), fermented, dried, and aged foods (including cured meats, green tea, Parmesan cheese, soy sauce, and balsamic vinegar), and also in the food additive MSG. Many classic food combinations maximize umami: Parmesan with tomato sauce, french fries with ketchup. (Breast milk apparently also has a relatively strong umami taste.)

WHAT YOU'LL NEED:
¼ teaspoon sugar or substitute of your choice (sweet)
¼ teaspoon sea salt (salty)
1 slice fresh lemon (sour)

1 small chunk unsweetened chocolate (e.g. Baker's brand) or 1 thin slice lemon peel (bitter)
1 thin slice Parmesan cheese (umami)
A glass of water

WHAT TO DO:

Sample the different tastes. Place each of the five different food samples on a plate in front of your child. Place an identical plate in front of yourself. Make sure you each have a glass of water to rinse your mouth with in between each sample. Start with whichever sample your child is most interested in trying. One by one, taste each sample. (If your child is reluctant to taste anything, don't worry. Ask them to simply touch each sample with their tongue—putting a bit on a spoon helps.)

Discuss what you've tasted. Encourage your child to name the tastes. Your child will probably be surprised by the bitter taste of the unsweetened chocolate. Discuss why chocolate normally tastes sweet, and how sugar masks the bitter taste.

Chat about tastes at mealtimes. Remind your child of the different tastes when they encounter them at mealtimes; for example, discuss "sour" tastes if you serve grapefruit in a fruit salad. Encourage your child to incorporate "sweet," "salty," "sour," "bitter," and "umami" into their descriptions of tastes, foods, and meals. You'll find that your child's perceptions will start to change; for example, they may start to think of sour as an "interesting" rather than "yucky" taste.

Game 3: Tasty Taste Buds (Ages 4 and Up)

MAIN MESSAGE:

We're able to taste food because of our taste buds (the tiny bumps on our tongues and in our mouths). Taste buds are just like muscles: they can be trained. And some are weaker (or stronger) than others.

WHAT YOU'LL NEED:

A mirror
A magnifying glass

WHAT TO DO:

Look at your tongue. Ask your child to look at their tongue in a mirror (a magnifying mirror, like those used for shaving, is great if you have it). Even better: have your child use a magnifying glass to look at your tongue or another family member's tongue. Ask your child to notice how the top of the tongue is bumpy and a bit rough-looking. Compare it to the underside, which is smoother. Explain that the bumps hold our taste buds. Older kids might be interested in the scientific word: papillae (*puh-PILL-ay*). The sandpaper-like texture of papillae also helps to grip food and move it around while we chew.

Young children can have up to 10,000 taste buds. Babies are born with more taste buds than adults and can taste what their mother has been eating—even before birth. As we age, our taste buds slowly atrophy, and the number of taste buds decreases. So, teenagers have fewer taste buds than young children, and adults have fewer than teenagers. This is why some foods may taste stronger to children than to adults.

Look more closely at your taste buds. Now that you both know what they look like, ask your child to look at their taste buds in a mirror. Have them drink a bit of milk, then look again. Can they see their taste buds more clearly? Ask your child to point out where their taste buds are the biggest and smallest, and whether some areas of their tongue have more taste buds than others. Some people have many more taste buds than others (these people are sometimes called "supertasters"—see Game 4: The Supertaster Game). Ask siblings and parents to drink a little milk and then have your child examine their taste buds, and then their own. Does one person seem to have more taste buds?

Try cooling your tongue (for ages 5 and up). Now that your child knows what taste buds look like, it's time to start learning more about how they work. Cold foods and drinks can make taste buds less sensitive. Cold can literally numb your taste buds: if you suck on an ice cube before you eat a food you don't like, you won't notice the taste as much. Try having your child taste a lemon—sour! Then ask them to put their tongue in a very cold glass of ice water or to suck on a plain ice popsicle for a few seconds. Have your child taste the lemon again. Does it taste less sour than before? Talk about why: just like cold fingers can't feel as well, cold taste buds are less sensitive.

A variation on this theme is to use a popsicle. Have your child try a sip of their favorite juice and then taste a popsicle made from that same juice (if possible, make your own with a home popsicle set, using the same juice). The frozen popsicle won't taste as sweet as the juice itself at room temperature.

Game 4: The Supertaster Game (Ages 6 and Up)

MAIN MESSAGE:

People are naturally more or less sensitive to tastes (see page 22 for a description of the three categories of tasters). In this game, your child will compare their taste buds (or, more precisely, the tiny bumps or papillae that house the taste buds on the tongue) with those of other people. The more papillae a person has, the more taste buds they have, and the more sensitive to taste they generally are. Kids will discover if they are more or less sensitive tasters, and that it may take more or less time for them to learn to like new foods, depending on which category of taster they fall into. Supertaster kids will feel reassured that it's natural for them to take a bit longer.

WHAT YOU'LL NEED:

Food coloring (green or blue works best)
Cotton swabs
Reinforcement rings for hole-punched paper (one per participant)
Magnifying glass

WHAT TO DO:

Guess your taste sensitivity. Tell your child you'll be doing a fun experiment. Explain that you'll be comparing the number of taste buds each of you have on your tongue using food coloring. Since the papillae don't absorb the food coloring, they remain red or pinkish (or even slightly whitish) in color, which makes it easier for kids to count the dots on their tongues. Explain to your child that you'll be using a simple measuring device (a reinforcement ring for hole-punched paper). On average, lower sensitivity tasters will have fewer than 15 papillae within the small circle, while supertasters may have twice that amount. Average tasters will be somewhere in the middle. Ask your child to guess whether they are an "average taster," a "supertaster," or a "low-sensitivity taster." (For younger children, you can just ask them to guess whether they'll have a "little," "average" or "middle," or "a lot.")

Count your taste buds. After you have recorded your child's guess, use a cotton swab to apply some food coloring onto your child's tongue. Place a reinforcement ring on the colored area and count the raised reddish/pink dots within the ring. Note: you are actually counting the papillae, on which the (much) smaller taste buds—which can't be seen by the naked eye—are clustered. Use a magnifying glass to help you. Double-count to check for accuracy. If you're really keen, you can compare the left and right sides of the tongue. Chances are that you'll have a lower number of papillae than the child—particularly on the tip of your tongue. Interestingly, conventional wisdom used to be that distinct regions of the tongue were sensitive to different tastes (for example, the tongue is most sensitive to salt at the front, to sweet on the sides near the front, and to sour on the sides near the back). However, researchers have recently revisited—and are hotly debating—this issue. The only point on which they currently seem to agree is that all areas of the tongue are somewhat sensitive to all of the tastes.

Chat about it. Your child will have lots of questions about this experiment. Here are a few questions you might ask: Was your prediction correct? What would happen if you had fewer taste buds—would food taste less strong? What if you had more taste buds: would you be more sensitive? Is this why it takes longer for sensitive tasters to get used to eating new foods? Ask your child to list some positive aspects of each type of taster. For example, non-tasters will get used to new foods easily and are less likely to be bothered by new foods when traveling. Supertasters might be able to detect whether food is spoiled more easily.

Top tips for learning to like new foods
- **Taste (and love of healthy foods) can be taught.** This is a basic skill that all children can learn.
- **Don't label your child a picky eater; they're "learning to like" new foods.** Remind your child that practice makes perfect. This is empowering for children, and calming for parents. With practice and repeated exposure, children can learn to appreciate lots of different foods. Tell this to your child—and remind yourself regularly! Your job is to make these foods available; your child's job is to gradually familiarize themselves with these foods. Some kids will take longer than others, so be patient.
- **For most children, pickiness is not a personality trait; it is a phase that they'll get over.** Neophobia—the universal fear of new foods that emerges around the

age of 2—is normal. Most children will go through a picky phase. *But this is only a phase.* Parents can help their child avoid this phase, or move through it more quickly, by helping them overcome their fear of new foods.

- **While all children can learn to eat a wide variety of foods, some will take longer than others** (just as some take longer to learn to read than others). There *are* differences between children. Some are generalized (for example, girls tend to have more taste buds than boys), and some are specific (for example, some children will truly have more sensitive taste buds than others). Be patient. Practice makes perfect.

- **Introduce your child to new foods before you serve them.** When children say "I don't like that food," they often mean "I don't know it." Showing them the food prior to eating it helps increase familiarity, and thus acceptance.

- **Take "no" for an answer if your child has had one bite.** If you use force or pressure, it will backfire. Be as calm as possible and make sure to offer the food again another day.

- **It's important to start young, if you can.** Beyond making it an easier process, researchers now suggest that dieting and eating disorders—which have been viewed as problems that emerge during adolescence—are also influenced by events prior to puberty, linked to parents' own eating habits, weight issues, and parental child-feeding practices.

- **It's not too late if your child is older.** The taste-training games are a fun way to help your child become more familiar with foods and help them understand their physical reactions. The recipes in the second half of the book are designed as a "ladder" to help your child move from simple to complex tastes and textures, and to tame new foods along the way.

- **Believe that your child can learn to eat, and like, all kinds of food.** Expect your child to develop more adventurous tastes and—eventually—they will, particularly if you model this yourself. This can take time, so be patient.

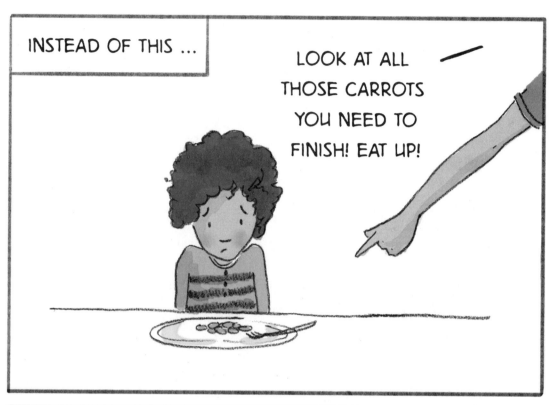

INSTEAD OF THIS ...

LOOK AT ALL THOSE CARROTS YOU NEED TO FINISH! EAT UP!

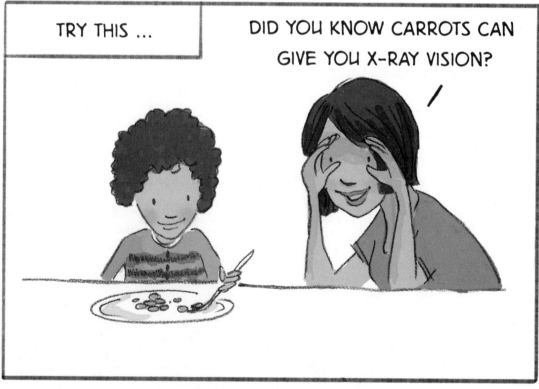

TRY THIS ...

DID YOU KNOW CARROTS CAN GIVE YOU X-RAY VISION?

SECRET 2

Marketing Healthy Food to Your Kids Really Works

Does yogurt grow on trees? Do sheep make eggs?

I N A RECENT SURVEY OF 1000 BRITISH PRIMARY SCHOOL STUDENTS, fewer than 1 in 4 knew that beef burgers came from cattle. Some said that eggs came from sheep. Others said that cheese came from butterflies. Fewer than 2 in 3 knew that potato chips are made with potatoes. Admittedly, these kids were relatively young. But even older children were found to have similar beliefs (my favorite: only 1 in 3 British teenagers correctly identified the sources of bacon, eggs, and milk). Studies in Australia yielded comparable results: when asked where yogurt came from, 1 in 4 Australian children thought it grew on trees. When shown a drawing of a lunch box with bread, cheese, and a banana, less than half of Australian students could identify all three items as coming from farms. One in 5 thought pasta came from an animal.

These examples are symptoms of food illiteracy: kids simply don't recognize an appropriate variety of foods, especially fruits and vegetables. More worryingly, even if children do have a high level of food and nutritional knowledge, they're not eating as well as they should.

The good news is that children can acquire food literacy pretty easily. Celebrity chef Jamie Oliver found this out while filming his hit TV show *Food Revolution* at a school in West Virginia. During one episode, a smiling Jamie places a bag on a desk in front of the kindergarteners, pulling vegetables out one by one. It's a cute scene, but something troubling quickly becomes apparent: the kids have no idea what *any* of the vegetables are. For cauliflower, one child bravely guesses "broccoli?" When shown a beet, the class is perplexed—another child ventures "celery?" Other children suggest that the eggplant Jamie proffers is a turnip, or a pear. A series of increasingly more desperate *"What's this?"* questions from Jamie culminates in the scene's climax: he holds up a bunch of ripe tomatoes. Surely, the kids will know what these are? After a painful silence, one brave child raises his hand and asks, "Are those potatoes?" Jamie then shows them two potatoes, and the class falls silent. "We use potatoes to make french fries, did you know that?" he asks. "No!" reply the children, most shaking their heads. In the scene's (depressing) finale, Jamie pulls out boxes of chicken nuggets, pizza, french fries, and hamburgers. The kids all give immediate, enthusiastic replies—they know exactly what these foods are (and it's clear that they like them).

The look on the teacher's face says it all. Her students have failed a test that she didn't even know she should have been preparing them for. The bad news is this is not unusual. But the good news is that kids can learn—and quickly. A few days later, Jamie went back to the classroom. This time, the kids shout out the answers cheerfully—and correctly.

Why is "getting to know" your vegetables important? Because eating well, as chef Cyril Lignac (France's answer to Jamie Oliver) says, requires that children "tame" new vegetables. In other words, they need to familiarize themselves, sort of like getting to know a new friend. The importance of familiarity—and the time it takes to develop it—is a key food education tactic. Often when kids say "I don't like it," they mean "I don't know it." Your job (as a parent or educator) is to help them get to know those new foods—to become food literate. Once children have got to know these foods, healthy eating will follow more easily.

Food literacy has two aspects: (1) Food knowledge: children are able to recognize a wide variety of foods and enjoy a wide variety of tastes. (2) Food awareness: children know where food comes from and how eating connects them to their families and communities. Without food literacy, our chances of countering the growing child obesity epidemic—which now affects not only wealthy countries, but also the majority of countries around the world—may be slim (no pun intended).

How food marketing undermines food literacy

OUR ABILITY TO TEACH OUR CHILDREN TO LOVE HEALTHY FOOD HAS BEEN increasingly undermined by food marketing, which is now a multi-billion dollar industry, using techniques that have become increasingly sophisticated. American kids are exposed to over 40,000 food ads per year—most of which are for fast food, cereal, and candy. And these ads work: marketing has a measurable effect on increasing consumption (if it didn't, why would those food companies spend all of that money?).

The message isn't only on TV, which is just the tip of the iceberg. Celebrity endorsements, product placement, discount pricing, and increased container sizes are all used to encourage increased consumption. Those candy bars at the checkout in your local grocery store? Chances are that a food company has paid the supermarket to place them there, right at kids' eye level.

Food advertising has also moved online in a big way, as it's both cheaper and a means of exposing kids to more advertising than on TV. The majority of top websites used by children contain food marketing. Other websites encourage kids to continue the "brand experience" after leaving the site (through screensavers or desktop logos). Food companies also use "adver-gaming," blurring the boundaries between games and advertising. In the game "Jell-O Jiggle It," kids can get a cube of Jell-O to dance. "Sour Fling" asks them to fling virtual Sour Patch Kids candies past obstacles. Or players can "lick" virtual lollipops in "Dum Dums Flick-A-Pop" (originally designed as "Lick-A-Pop," before Apple complained that iPhones could be damaged by too much saliva); the app has been downloaded 1.5 million times. A step up in complexity is "Candy Sports," in which players can hit baseballs at a Skittles logo, play basketball in an arena plastered with Life Savers Gummies, and kick footballs into a Starburst sign. The self-explanatory "Cookie Dough Bites Factory" has been downloaded more than 3 million times.

Full-blown websites have more complex games, such as Nestlé's "Nesquik Imagination Station" (hosted by a cute rabbit character, with a quiz game and spacesuit-making guide) or the imaginary McWorld on HappyMeals.com (complete with treehouse games for younger kids—pick your own Mc-Avatar!—and a sci-fi movie and book series for older kids). HappyMeals.com had 350,000 visitors in *one single month* in 2011.

Marketers also target adolescents on popular social media sites (like Facebook and Twitter), via smartphones and viral marketing (such as videos meant to be shared with friends), and even through sophisticated techniques like downloadable widgets (small applications downloaded to a child's computer or phone that allow companies to deliver targeted ads to users and their friends). Many of these approaches target older children's and adolescents' developmental needs—such as bonding with peers and establishing their own identity—and are thus hard to resist, which makes them potentially more dangerous than traditional forms of advertising because they seek to elicit emotional responses and hence deep loyalty to brands.

Of course, marketing is a legitimate business activity. If it encourages children to overeat unhealthy foods, however, it has both health and economic implications—particularly (although not only) obesity-related. This issue is now of such concern to policy-makers that the United States Congress recently asked the top medical research agency in the country—the Center for Disease Control and Prevention—to study the link between obesity and food marketing to children. The resulting Institute of Medicine study, *Food Marketing to Children and Youth: Threat or Opportunity,* makes for chilling reading. The report found that food marketing intentionally targets children who are too young to distinguish between truth and advertising. Researchers now believe that the effects of marketing on our subconscious, automatic behaviors are widespread and long lasting. By watching these ads, our children may literally be programmed for a lifetime of unhealthy eating.

The report also documents the tactics used by food marketing companies to make their messages compelling. Food marketing companies conduct extensive research on children—even preschoolers. To improve their ability to leverage children's suggestibility, they explore the psychological underpinnings of children's food choices, probing and testing "child archetypes" (to get their spokes-characters just right), and figuring out ways to help kids leverage or subvert the "psyche of mothers as the family gatekeeper." Marketing strategies have proliferated, and got subtler, targeting "cool" messages at some age groups and "cute" messages at others, until heavily marketed brands become central to children's sense of identity and self. Scary.

Of course, marketers argue that advertising is free speech and that marketing is good for business. Those same arguments were used for cigarette marketing in the past—and are arguments we should no longer accept, as Marion Nestle has brilliantly argued in her book *Food Politics*. But the power of the food industry is such that the regulatory controls that exist in some countries—like France, where vending machines, fast food, and food advertising of any kind are banned in all schools—are far from universal.

So what's a parent to do? Of course, you can reduce your kids' exposure to marketing messages. Even simply setting limits on screen time has been shown to be beneficial for kids' health. This is, in part, because exposure to TV food advertising (with its "snacking = enjoyment" messages) increases calories consumed during and immediately afterward—whether or not kids are actually hungry. (This is true for adults, too, by the way.)

I realize that turning off the TV isn't likely to make you a popular parent. Luckily, there are positive things you can do. One of the most powerful strategies of all turns marketing on its head: *you* can market food to your kids.

You can market food to your kids!

CORNELL UNIVERSITY MARKETING GURU BRIAN WANSINK HAS SPENT decades finding ways to market healthy food to kids. His idea is simple: Why not invert the logic of food marketers, which masterfully induces cravings for processed foods and junk foods of all kinds? This sounded like a tall task: how could academic researchers, no matter how savvy, take on marketing companies with million-dollar advertising budgets?

Wansink's strategy was ingenious in its simplicity. He found that renaming vegetables with silly (or branded) names worked wonders with kids. His team served "X-ray Vision Carrots" and "Power Punch Broccoli," along with "Tiny Tasty Tree Tops" and "Silly Dilly Green Beans." They tested this out in a few schools (including two in New York) with amazing results: up to 100 percent increased consumption of vegetables. Another experiment by Wansink's team found that preschoolers were more likely to make healthy choices if foods were visually branded with sympathetic figures (as simple as an Elmo sticker on an apple).

Wansink also developed an experiment for older kids, specifically focused on healthy choices in fast food restaurants. This is admittedly a tough nut to crack: even though many fast food restaurants now offer healthy choices, few kids pick them. Realistically, how many kids are going to choose a side salad instead of fries (even if offered Newman's Own Balsamic Vinaigrette)? And would apple dippers really beat out a vanilla ice-cream cone? Not for most kids.

Wansink was convinced that something *could* be done to help kids make healthy choices. His research team designed an experiment that would prime kids through the power of suggestion and association. The experiment was simple: kids at a summer camp, ranging from 6 to 12 years old, were asked to participate in the study. They were invited to go out for a fast food lunch once per week, 4 weeks in a row. (I'm thinking it wasn't very hard to convince kids to sign up for this experiment.)

At each lunch, each child was given a choice between french fries and apple dippers. The first week, kids were simply asked what they wanted, without any attempt to influence their choices. The second week, however, kids were asked to complete a brief questionnaire, privately, before going to the restaurant. Researchers showed each child pictures of six superheroes and asked them what the superhero would eat: apples or fries? Kids were then asked what their own choice would be. The next week, kids were shown several pictures of healthy foods (including fries and apples), and then were asked to classify the foods as healthy or unhealthy. Again, after the exercise, the kids were asked to choose between french fries and apple dippers. The result? In the first week, only 1 in 10 kids picked the apple slices. After being asked about superhero choices, nearly 5 out of 10 children (*half* the kids) picked apples.

I appreciated Wansink's insights when we were over at my cousin's house for dinner one night. A fairly zealous whole foods sort of person (without kids), she had prepared a wonderful dinner that featured braised kale and pearl barley. As she proudly served them, my daughters stared at their plates for a few seconds while I watched, wondering what to do (they'd never had pearl barley before). Meanwhile, the smell of the barley—a yeasty fresh-bread-just-out-of-the-oven sort of smell—wafted over the table.

"It smells like bread!" exclaimed Claire. I had my eureka moment.

"What's that?" Sophie cautiously asked, fidgeting and ever so slowly sliding her plate away from her.

"Oh, that's Fairy Baguette," I said cheerfully, sliding the plate back toward her. "Fairies are tiny, and this is like mini-bread just their size."

Sophie looked dubious, but Claire took the bait.

"Fairy Baguette? Yum!" she chirped, before picking up a grain of barley and nibbling on it. "It's delicious. Try some!" And her older sister did just that.

Of course, you don't have to use only child-friendly names to work your marketing magic. The French tend to use place-based names for dishes. Often, those names relate to the places where the food is from, with a regional *terroir* ("taste of place") emphasis that is so characteristic of French family cuisine. Vicious Carrots (see page 189) is a divine, melt-in-your-mouth carrot dish (and super easy to make) that conjures up images of traditional cuisine in one of France's heartlands. Or think of the classic beef bourguignon, which comes from Burgundy, southeast of Paris, one of the gastronomic heartlands of France. Or what about the dessert favorite *Poires Belle Hélène* (see page 279), invented by renowned chef Escoffier, named after a 19th-century opera by Offenbach. This is the equivalent of naming a dish after a blockbuster movie. Avatar Asparagus? Harry Potter Hash Browns? Lion King Lettuce? You get the idea.

The take-home message is simple: appealing names work wonders. Families often find that this is a nice alternative to the sneaky chef method: renaming foods (rather than hiding them) allows kids to get over their food fears. One of our French friends, Virginie, loves to tell the story about "sea chicken" (*poule de mer*). Her older daughter Emma didn't like fish, but loved chicken. So Virginie hit on the idea of serving relatively mild, white fish (like sole) and calling it "sea chicken." It took years before Emma liked fish, but she never once balked at her *poule de mer* dish.

Another simple experiment one of my test families tried was with potatoes. Kristine's 2- and 5-year-old girls refused to eat potatoes, flat out. They'd been that way since they started solids. I suggested something that I'd tried when my younger daughter, Claire, balked at eating potatoes: renaming them "volcanoes." The approach is simple: mash up a boiled potato into a cone shape, poke a small hole in the top, stick a little piece of butter in the top, and watch the butter melt and run down the sides like (you guessed it) lava. Here's what Kristine had to say:

> On your advice, at Thanksgiving dinner I mounded the potatoes, made a hole in the top, and poured in the gravy, then told the girls in an excited tone that they were eating "potato volcanoes." The girls ate every bite. This idea is pure genius.
>
> —KRISTINE

The power of parent-led marketing

ONE OF THE MOST POWERFUL WAYS TO MARKET FOOD TO CHILDREN IS TO USE parental role modeling. If parents (or other trusted caregivers) are seen to eat a food and enjoy it, kids are much more likely to try it and to report that they liked it. This parental effect was even more pronounced with younger children. The families that offered new foods in a loving, calm environment achieved the best results. In one experiment, children were given the option of eating a sandwich with a new and unfamiliar filling alone or while sitting with their mother and having a quiet but social time together. Children who chose the latter option (and the majority did) not only liked the new filling more at the end of the six-week experiment, they were also more likely to try other new foods.

My test families report that teaching children to like new foods often means that parents have to change their cooking and eating habits. Remember 3-year-old Lucas? When his parents began taste training, his mother, Jessica, realized that it might help if she started to do some of the cooking (her husband had been doing most of it). "I realized that the reason the only meat Lucas liked to eat was hot dogs was that it was the only kind of meat I felt comfortable cooking," she confessed. With encouragement from her husband, Jessica tried out a variety of easy vegetable recipes (all included in the second part this book) and found—to her delight—that there are vegetables Lucas actually loves, including ones that Jessica herself had trouble eating as a child. Most important, reports Jessica, "I think it's great that Lucas sees his mom in the kitchen—it helps to illustrate how important food is to us, and how much we enjoy it."

The Me Too Method

ONE OF THE FUN TWISTS ON PARENT-LED MARKETING IS SOMETHING I CALL the "Me Too Method." The idea is simple: if you serve it to yourself and eat it with obvious enjoyment, children's natural curiosity will be piqued, and they'll be more likely to want some, too. I've tried this numerous times in the past but recently decided to test this method again one night. After our main course, I served myself some lovely baby spinach salad, topped with vinaigrette and tiny little pieces of mandarin orange. I didn't say a word to the kids, but calmly kept chatting to my husband about our day. My younger daughter, Claire—who is not the world's most enthusiastic salad eater—looked up at me and said, "Why didn't *I* get any salad?" Sophie, never one to like being left out, followed suit. They both promptly proceeded to eat a plateful of salad.

Christine, one of my readers, used this approach to great effect with her toddler, who was having a hard time learning to like yogurt. In fact, Christine barely had time to put yogurt down on the table before the "no yogurt!" refrain would be heard. One day she decided to try something different. Instead of a plastic tub, Christine put a new, small glass bowl on the table. "Look! Look at your beautiful new tasting bowl!" Her toddler examined it with great intrigue and watched as Christine placed a dollop of pink (raspberry) yogurt into it, saying, "Here's a tiny taste for you." Christine then proceeded to eat a spoonful of her own, savoring it with lots of "mmmm" and "yum," obviously relishing the sweet taste. After a moment, her toddler grabbed her own spoon and popped a bit of yogurt into her mouth. Then, with obvious delight, the little hand darted out again and again, until she cleaned her bowl. "I took a taste!" was her proud response. Now yogurt is a favorite in Christine's house.

The "why" of eating: It's not about nutrition

MARKETING FOOD TO YOUR KIDS ISN'T JUST A PLAYFUL DISTRACTION. IT'S actually a crucial contribution to their eating success. Research shows that food *preferences* (not nutritional knowledge) play a crucial role in enabling children (and adults) to make healthy food choices. In other words, we eat what we *like* to eat, even if we know it's not good for us. We avoid eating what we don't like to eat, even if we know it *is* good for us.

In fact, nutritional information can backfire. Dr. Marion Nestle argues that many of us suffer from nutrition confusion: conflicting, competing, and rapidly changing nutrition claims that confuse consumers, increase anxiety, and encourage us to buy over-processed foods on the basis of (at times) dubious nutritional claims. Because of this, many nutritionists now recommend a different, simpler idea: the greater variety of foods (including fruits and vegetables) a child eats, the wider range of nutrients they will get.

Your goal is to get your child eating a variety of foods. Marketing healthy foods to your child helps them establish the right food preferences. If you just worry about nutrition, you're fighting a losing battle. Instead of telling your child "Eat this, it's good for you," try telling them "Eat this, it tastes good!"

> At dinner tonight, instead of saying "You have to eat this," I kept saying "Yum, it's delicious!" My 3-year-old kept laughing and repeating it—and ate her entire dinner without a complaint. I'm not exaggerating—she's really changed her approach overnight.
>
> —FRANÇOISE

In other words, *telling* your child to eat a variety of foods so that they get nutrients isn't a great strategy for success. Enabling them to eat these foods because they truly believe they are yummy will, for most kids, work better. And vitamins and minerals are better absorbed from fresh food than from vitamin pills. When I asked our family doctor in France whether Claire was getting enough iron and needed iron supplements, he looked at me curiously and then laughed. "Get her to eat parsley and beets" was his calm response.

I'll admit that getting children to eat a variety of nutrient-rich foods often requires parents to be inventive—but it can also be fun. I remember the time our friends Sonja and Jamie visited us with their daughter, Carrie, a feisty 2-year-old and rigidly picky eater who at that time was eating only scrambled eggs and buttered toast—for breakfast, lunch, and dinner. Despite their efforts, green vegetables in any form would not pass this child's lips.

"She won't eat anything but scrambled eggs," her mother told us, evidently consigned to her child's fate (with Carrie in the room, who was quietly, but intently, listening). "You want to bet?" replied my husband, Philippe, who took this on as a personal challenge. After a bit of brainstorming, he took some of the rice we had cooked for dinner and mixed it in the food processor with some steamed spinach and a big dollop of honey. He poured the velvety smooth, melt-in-your-mouth, electric green purée into a little bowl with a cheerful cartoon on the bottom. Tiny dabs of butter decorated the top: two eyes, a nose, and a little button mouth.

"Look what we're eating! Spinach Surprise!" announced Philippe, with just a little bit of a flourish. As he handed the bowl to Carrie he said in a firm, inviting voice, "There's a *surprise* at the bottom of *your* bowl—but only yours!" The rest of us were handed normal white bowls, and we dipped our spoons in without comment (her parents having been instructed to say nothing and to continue our dinner conversation as if nothing out of the ordinary was happening).

At first, Carrie looked mutinous. She stared at her bowl. Her bowl stared back at her. (As instructed, we all stared at our bowls, too, and then started eating.)

"Quick—the eye is melting!" joked my husband. He popped Carrie's spoon into the bowl, nestling it just under the dab of butter in question—which now looked quite teary-eyed, as the butter melted in a little transparent yellow streak. He turned away to continue his conversation.

Out of the corner of my eye, I saw Carrie take a quick look around the table, scowling. Not getting any attention, her eyes strayed to her bowl. After a minute's hesitation, she tentatively lifted the spoon to her mouth and oh-so-delicately licked the teeniest, tiniest bit of buttery spinach. Thoughtfully, she licked her lips, casting her eyes around the table. Nobody, it seemed, was paying attention. Then the spoon reached down for the other "eye." And then the nose, then the mouth . . . until Carrie had scraped the bowl clean and found the cartoon hiding at the bottom of her bowl.

Carrie is now a healthy, athletic teenager who eats pretty much everything (including spinach). How did she get there? First, lots of practice. Her parents exposed her to vegetables over and over again, in lots of different ways. Second, creativity: they figured out which recipes, cooking strategies, and presentation (including fun names) worked best for their family. Third, they made family meals fun.

Note that I didn't mention nutritional information. Do you really think that a toddler who can't yet count to 100 is going to be motivated to eat their spinach because it's "high in iron"? You know that your kids should eat certain foods, but using nutritional information to encourage them is probably not going to work. (In fact, it doesn't really work for most adults either.)

Tactics to avoid: When marketing backfires

MARKETING FOOD TO KIDS WORKS BEST WHEN YOU ADOPT A POSITIVE approach. When you market healthy foods to your children, emphasize pleasure rather than the deprivation associated with diets or banning certain foods.

You can also teach your kids to seek out good foods that they enjoy (which I call "eat most of the time foods") rather than avoiding "bad" foods (which you can label "once in a while foods"). Try to avoid making your child feel guilty for enjoying treats. Avoiding negative emotional associations with food helps children avoid feelings of guilt that might translate into emotional eating and poor eating habits, and even eating disorders. After all, treats are fun—in moderation.

Although being positive is important, don't overdo the praise. A degree of praise can increase how much children perceive they enjoy (and actually consume) healthy foods, but too much praise can make children uncomfortable or even backfire. Simple yet positive observations ("You enjoyed your meal, didn't you?" or "You did your best at tasting that new food") will make a child more comfortable than lavish praise, which might imply blame or parental anxiety if the child doesn't measure up.

Perhaps most important, don't use bribes or rewards. Research shows that these increase kids' preferences for the "reward" food (such as dessert) and decrease their preferences for the "required" food (such as salad). Bribes and rewards might work in the short term, but they don't teach kids the right behaviors in the long term.

Marketing food to your kids: Getting started

HOW CAN YOU PUT THESE MARKETING IDEAS INTO ACTION? IN ADDITION TO the ideas discussed in this chapter, here are four fun games that will teach your kids important concepts—such as how our sense of smell is related to taste—and will give you some surefire strategies for taking the fear out of new foods.

Game 5: The Silly Name Game (Ages 3 and Up)

MAIN MESSAGE:

This fun game involves labeling foods with names that will ignite your child's enthusiasm for new foods. Using "superhero" or "silly" names might work for younger kids; stylish or "cool" names might work for older kids.

In case you're dubious, let me reassure you: everyone who has tried this game has told me that it works. Parents have so few fun, easy tactics in their arsenal that you shouldn't pass this one up. Moreover, there's a difference between being playful and playing with food. In the former case, you can be respectful of the food but still light-hearted about it. This doesn't mean you allow kids to actually play with their food. Rather, you focus on putting them in a relaxed (rather than oppositional) mood, which makes mealtime easier. Remember that renaming strange foods in ways that make them familiar can help your kids get over the fear of new foods, making it easier for them to adapt (particularly when you're traveling or eating at other people's houses).

WHAT YOU'LL NEED:

Imagination and a sense of humor

WHAT TO DO:

Ask your child to name dishes (or name dishes in their honor if they help design or make them). If you travel, try to sample at least one local dish; when you're back home, try making it and give it a name that refers to the place where you first ate it. Or try silly names—even with older kids. You might be surprised by how much they enjoy it.

When I asked other parents about the Silly Name Game, I got some great suggestions. Turns out that lots of parents already do this. Nina wrote to me to tell me that spinach is called Monster Surprise in her house. When introducing broccoli to her toddler, Brandy explained that broccoli buds were baby flower buds—and her toddler promptly renamed it "Broccoli Flowers," which she ate with gusto.

You can also use the power of association. You can apply this logic when eating out, using your child's favorite superhero (or just plain hero!). "What would Batman pick?" was used in the experiment described earlier in this chapter. "What would Dora pick?" would work in my younger daughter's case. Or, for older kids, pick a sports figure or celebrity—or someone you know personally who they look up to—who's known for healthy eating.

Game 6: The Smell-Taste Experiment (Ages 6 and Up)

MAIN MESSAGE:

This game teaches kids that our senses of smell and taste are related. It also helps them understand that smell plays a large part in determining how things taste. Kids will even learn how artificial flavors are used to fool our taste buds (the most fun part of this game).

WHAT YOU'LL NEED:

3 lollipops of different flavors (but similar textures)
A blindfold

WHAT TO DO:

Discuss the relationship between smell and taste. Ask your child to think about how smell and taste may be related. For example, ask your child if they have ever noticed how having a cold diminishes their sense of taste. Explain this is because their sense of smell is temporarily affected. For older children, you can explain the relationship between smell and taste in a bit more detail. Aromas are detected when odors (airborne molecules) pass through the nose and are absorbed by cells inside the nose. When the nose is blocked, the tongue will taste the sugar and acid, but not detect the lemon smell, for example. Smell thus enhances the taste of food by allowing us to combine complex aromas with the five basic tastes. Older kids may also enjoy learning new vocabulary. The word "olfaction" refers to our sense of smell. The word "gustation" refers to our sense of taste.

Plug your nose. Blindfold your child, ask them to plug their nose, and have them try each flavored lollipop, one after the other. Ask them to guess the flavor of each lollipop. This is way more difficult than you might expect.

Chat about flavors. Ask your child why they think food companies would use artificial flavors in food. You can explain that many artificial foods (such as candies) are made from similar ingredients and so have very similar tastes, and that it is the use of different scents or perfumes that makes them taste different. Many food companies employ flavorists (yes, this is a real job) to create these smell/taste combinations using edible chemicals and extracts that alter the flavor of food through influencing our sense of smell.

Game 7: The Mystery Smell Game (Ages 6 and Up)

MAIN MESSAGE:

This game introduces the idea that smells have strong emotional associations and often help us recall memories of places, people, or events. Children will experience how smell evokes memories and emotions and connect this to their feelings about food.

WHAT YOU'LL NEED:

A blindfold

Cotton balls

Containers, preferably plastic ones with lids

4 or 5 items with scents, including:

- Familiar smells (for example: perfume, shampoo, vanilla extract, lemon, banana, cinnamon)
- Pungent smells (for example: pine needles, vinegar, coffee, ginger, garlic, peppermint, curry powder)
- Hard-to-identify smells (for example: pencil shavings, dirt, olive oil, a slice of raw potato, a slice of raw cabbage)

WHAT TO DO:

Prepare the containers. Place a different item in each container (for liquids, soak a cotton ball and place that in the container). Keep the items separated and the containers closed to prevent the odors from mixing.

Smell the items. Ask your child to put on the blindfold and then smell the containers one by one. Then ask your child to rate the odor: older kids can use more complex language ("strong," "neutral," "pleasant," "pungent"); younger kids can simply say "good" or "bad."

Chat about it. Ask your child if they think a substance is edible or not (regardless of whether they correctly identify it). Ask your child to talk about any memories associated with the smells. You might be surprised by the responses. You can give your own examples (one brand of shampoo reminds me of summer camp, and a specific type of perfume always reminds me of my mom).

Game 8: The Store-Brand versus Name-Brand Blind Taste Test (Ages 9 and Up)

MAIN MESSAGE:

Brands influence our perception of taste and quality. Even if the food doesn't taste better, our belief that it will (which is created by the branding) influences our sense of taste. This game helps children to think critically about their emotional responses to branding.

WHAT YOU'LL NEED:

Pick at least two matching pairs of name-brand and store-brand items. Here's a list of potential pairs, taken from a *Consumer Reports* test of name-brand/store-brand pairs:

- Kellogg's Rice Krispies versus store-brand rice cereal
- Skippy peanut butter versus store-brand peanut butter
- Nature's Valley granola bars versus store-brand granola bars
- Coca-Cola or Pepsi versus store-brand cola
- Wonder Bread versus store-brand bread
- Minute Maid versus store-brand orange juice

WHAT TO DO:

Chat about branding. Ask your child whether they think that brands influence their sense of taste. With older children, you can discuss how branding influences taste. For example, in one study, kids liked the taste of foods more when they were presented in McDonald's packaging, compared with the identical foods without any branding. In another experiment, children were shown an enjoyable ad for a new food and then tried the food; they rated the new food tastier than those who tried the food before viewing the ad. Studies with teens and adults have shown similar effects, like the famous blind taste test for name-brand cola versus store-brand cola.

Sample the blinded pairs. Ask your child to sample each pair of products and record their observations (what they liked and didn't like) and overall preferences. At the end, reveal their preferences and count up the number of choices of name-brand versus store-brand options.

Variation: The Switcheroo

Switch the labels on the name-brand and store-brand products. For example, you would put out the following, clearly labeled:

- One bowl of Rice Krispies cereal (labeled "store brand") and one bowl of store-brand rice cereal (labeled "Rice Krispies")
- One glass of name-brand cola (labeled "store brand") and one glass of store-brand cola (labeled with the name brand)

Ask your child to taste both samples and indicate which one they prefer, then reveal the switch.

Chat about the results. Has your child ever pestered you for a name-brand product and resisted the store brand? Ask them to think about why.

If you did the "switcheroo" experiment and your child preferred the store brand in the name-brand packaging, ask them why they thought this was the case. How much did their belief about the brand influence their expectations and actual taste experience?

An important point to discuss with your child is how much more the name-brand products cost versus the store-brand products. A name-brand granola bar may be almost twice as expensive as a store-brand granola bar, for example. Is the extra money worth it? Why (or why not)?

Top Tips for Marketing Healthy Food to Your Kids

- **Talk less about health and more about good tastes.** Don't cajole with nutritional information (such as explanations that a food has a lot of iron or calcium). Instead, emphasize how delicious the food is. For example, try saying "Taste this, it's really yummy" rather than "Eat this, it's good for you." Tell your children that good-for-you foods taste good. Healthy eating habits will be a happy by-product. *"Broccoli? Yum!"*

- **Eat with your children, tasting foods with obvious enjoyment.** Are you modeling picky eating behavior for your children? If so, consider changing your own eating habits. Get other influential role models involved (like older peers) when possible.

- **Give dishes attractive (or silly) names.** Sound silly? The Silly Name Game (page 52) shows the contrary—it works, even on adults.

- **Don't use bribes or rewards.** Research shows that these increase kids' preferences for the "reward" food (such as dessert) and decrease their preferences for the "required" food (such as salad).

- **Do use moderate praise.** A recent study showed that social praise actually increased intrinsic liking for and consumption of healthy foods among children over a 3-month period. (But don't overdo it—it may backfire.)

- **Don't label foods as "good" or "bad."** Call foods "eat most of the time foods" and "occasional treats." Teach your child the difference, and don't make them feel guilty for enjoying treats—that way you'll avoid emotional eating.

- **Teach your kids to seek out good foods they enjoy (rather than avoiding "bad" foods).** The difference is subtle but important. Healthy eating is about pleasure, not deprivation.

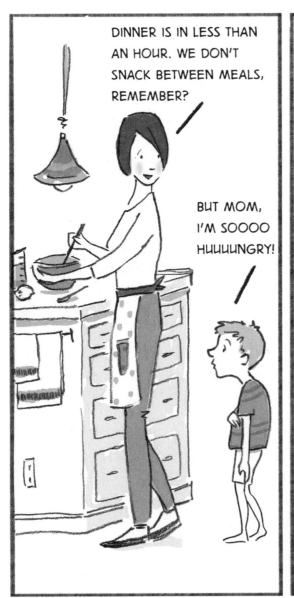

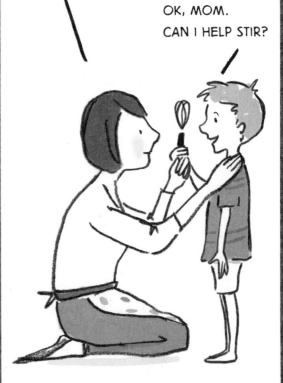

Schedule One Snack a Day

Ask a North American parent whether they pack food when leaving home with their kids, and chances are that they're hoarding snacks. Crackers, granola bars, juice boxes, dried cereal, and more are tucked away in pockets, purses, glove compartments, and bags for that inevitable moment when children declare they are hungry. The cozy, even comforting, image of snack-time is a cliché of childhood. Kids need to snack, right? Tiny tummies need filling up at regular intervals, right? Even if they didn't, the prospect of a food deprivation–induced tantrum is more than many parents can bear. Anyway, why would you deprive a child of their snack? With kids, it's normal that snack-time is pretty much all the time, isn't it?

Well, it turns out that this behavior is normal in North America but not (at least traditionally) in many other places. In China, snacking is rare, and foods consumed as snacks (such as rice crackers) are low in calories. In Italy, meals are eaten three times a day, with only one snack—a mid-afternoon snack called the *merenda*. The same is true in France, where children as young as 2 years old happily subsist on four meals a day: breakfast, lunch, dinner, and a scheduled afternoon snack (actually more like a mini-meal) known as the *goûter* (goo-*tay*). Of course, cultural norms for eating differ greatly from one country to the next, but it seems safe to say that prior to the advent of industrial food culture, snacking used to be relatively rare—both because of constraints (lack of income; the time and expense needed to gather and prepare foods; lack of ability to ship and store prepared foods) and folk wisdom about regulating one's eating habits.

The modern "snack-time all the time" phenomenon is, it turns out, relatively recent. Snacking rates rose rapidly from the 1970s onward, along with the rise of processed food and the food marketing industry. Back in the 70s, North American children snacked once a day (and a quarter of kids didn't snack at all). Today, North American kids snack on average three times a day; and one in five children snacks five times a day or more. (A significant proportion of adults also snack multiple times per day.) And they're not alone: children in many countries—from England to Australia to India to Mexico—have jumped on the snacking bandwagon.

The increase in snacking is one of the major causes of increasing child obesity rates. As much as we wish otherwise, most kids aren't chowing down on apples and carrots. Salty snacks, soda, and candy are the most popular choices—and biggest calorie jolts. Snacks are the source for more than 1 in 4 calories that our kids now consume. At the same time, fewer children are eating three regular meals per day. Snacks are substituting for breakfast or even lunch—with some schools even going so far as to replace lunchtime with "snack breaks" or "nutrition breaks" to save time during the school day.

However, most doctors and other medical experts argue that frequent snacking is a bad idea because kids often aren't hungry enough to eat the nutritious foods served at mealtimes. That's not all: since adult food habits are formed during childhood, excessive snacking teaches our kids poor eating habits. Feeding kids typical snack foods fosters taste preferences for poor-quality foods of little nutritional value. Most processed snack food is engineered to achieve precisely this result, with addictive combinations of fat, sugar, and salt that are designed to keep us coming back for more. Snacking leads us to overeat while (ironically) decreasing our overall intake of nutrients. Simply put: kids don't need to snack. They might *want* to, but they don't *need* to.

The assertion that kids don't need more than one snack per day is controversial. On the one hand, some parents argue that regular snacking has benefits (balancing out blood glucose levels, for example). Some snacking supporters argue that "grazing" (random snacking) is fine, as long as the foods being consumed are healthy. Other parents disagree. They argue that random snacking might be fine when your preschooler has a choice between cucumbers and carrots at home, but not so desirable when kids hit high school, with access to vending machines and fast food. Others argue that unrestricted snacking creates a deregulated approach to eating that might work for a toddler, but not as a lifelong approach to eating.

One fact seems clear: if eating any time or all the time becomes normal, children risk developing a habit of eating even when they aren't hungry. And if snacking is used to regulate children's behavior (in response to crankiness, for example), this creates the risk of allowing your child to develop emotional eating behaviors. Bored? Why not go to the cupboard and rummage around for some Fruit by the Foot? Tired? Here, have some Goldfish crackers.

The best way to avoid emotional eating is by scheduling meals and snacks; this takes emotions and impulsive eating out of the equation. That's not all: studies show that scheduling snacking reduces obesity rates. But what schedule will work best? Most experts recommend allowing children to snack at most twice a day (and preferably, for kids 6 and up, only once per day). Make sure to schedule three predictable, nutritious, filling meals per day. For children under 5, offer two snacks a day: one in mid-morning and one in mid-afternoon. For children 5 and older, offer one snack a day, usually in the mid- to late afternoon. This routine may evolve as your children grow, participate in sports, and so on. For teenagers, try increasing the size of their meals and snack rather than adding more snacks to their routine.

Many of my test families had great results by creating a snacking routine. Heidi wrote to me to explain how well this snacking routine was working for her family after I posted some ideas on my blog:

> *The snack thing has been way out of control in our house. I had never thought about the snacking as having any negative effects. We only offer healthy snacks, and the North American view that children need to eat frequently and that many small meals are healthier than three big ones had led me not to question the snacking habit. After deciding to follow the "one snack per day" approach, I tracked what the kids ate for a few days and realized they were eating much less protein and vegetables than I realized because of all the fruit, crackers, muffins, smoothies, and granola bars they were eating as snacks all day. Often the kids weren't hungry for dinner, ate only half of it, and then got more snacks later. The eating on the go, the crumbs, the mess, the snack containers going missing! We've now eliminated snacks to one substantial after-school snack, and it has made a huge difference in how much dinner the kids eat. They are also not hungry for bedtime snacks, either. I love this!*
>
> —HEIDI

Pediatrician Nimali Fernando, who blogs under the name "Doctor Yum," also wrote to me with her thoughts. Nimali confessed she wasn't different from most American moms. She carried snacks "just in case" (What if someone has a meltdown? What if the family is stuck somewhere without food?), and their kitchen counter featured a big snack basket, which her kids invariably dipped into right before dinner. Inspired by the "one snack per day" idea, Nimali tried her own experiment at home:

For the past month, I have instituted a "no snacking" and "le goûter" (afternoon snack) at my house, and I'm pleased to say it has worked brilliantly. During soccer season, our heartier goûter snack held the kids over until after practice, and the kids were much more able to eat a nutritious dinner that I served because they weren't munching in the car on the way home. The kids now understand the rules about snacking, and as long as they have plenty to do, they don't seem to miss snacks.

—NIMALI

Nimali and her family learned an important lesson: mild hunger is a normal human sensation. If children's (and adults') stomachs are comfortably empty before mealtimes, they will be more likely to eat well. As Nimali summed it up, "A child who is faced with broccoli at dinner is more likely to eat it if she's not full of fish crackers and fruit snacks."

Just like Doctor Yum, when my daughters tell me they feel hungry, I don't necessarily feed them. I check in with our routine. If it's not time to eat, I tell them, "That's great, you'll really appreciate your next meal. It's in X hours." Sometimes the next meal is only an hour away, but sometimes it is 2 or 3 hours away. That's okay—they know they have to wait. My kids and I both know that we have a set routine in our house: three nutritious, energy-dense meals a day (at which they can eat as much or as little as they want), and one ample afternoon snack. This means that they eat as much as they feel they need at meals, and know they will be able to eat well at their next meal.

The difference between feeling hungry and being hungry

DOCTOR YUM'S STORY RAISES AN IMPORTANT POINT: IT'S OKAY FOR YOUR child to feel a little bit hungry. If they eat three meals and one nutritious snack per day, your child will not starve. Research shows that children intuitively compensate by eating more at mealtimes (provided, of course, that those mealtimes are scheduled and predictable). By limiting snacks, you're enabling them to establish this internal regulation skill whereby they can sense whether they're hungry or not. And by permitting them to snack all the time (or by offering overly large portions or calorie-laden sweet or salty snack foods), you are undermining this skill.

No one wants a child to *be* hungry, but we seem to have extended the term "hungry" to include everything from feeling peckish to being malnourished. This is often associated with the habit of feeding kids as soon as (or even before) they let you know they're hungry. By doing so, parents miss an opportunity to teach their child a valuable skill: knowing what a comfortably empty stomach feels like. This skill allows children not to overeat and to wait comfortably until the next mealtime—a classic example of self-regulation.

How do you teach your child this approach? Simple: just don't let them randomly snack. If you do snack, schedule it. When you set up this schedule, explain to your child that "We only eat at mealtimes, and otherwise we can happily wait." Being happy with that feeling of a comfortably empty stomach will enable your child to wait patiently until their next meal—setting up good eating habits for life.

The French have an expression for this feeling of pre-meal hunger: they call it a *bonne maladie* (a "good illness"). This feeling, they tell their children, is a *good* feeling—kind of like that wonderful anticipation you feel in the run-up to your birthday. You wouldn't have your birthday party a week early, would you? There's nothing wrong with feeling a bit hungry if a nutritious and filling meal is going to be on the table soon.

Remember: don't feel panicked at the thought of your child feeling hungry (as opposed to truly *being* hungry). I know many parents might (I certainly did when we transitioned our daughters). One mom, Shaylagh, wrote to me about these fears. She confessed that she had become a "fear feeder," despite her best intentions. As Shaylagh noted, "I'd fill his belly to avoid conflict and then wonder why he was fussy at dinner." But after she established a meal and snack schedule, her toddler's behavior improved. No more negotiating, impulsiveness, or tantrums. Shaylagh had discovered one of the most helpful principles of parenting: children will behave well when the rules are known and followed consistently because they're confident their needs will be met in a timely and satisfying fashion.

The art of anticipation: Teaching patience

SCHEDULING SNACKS IS A GREAT WAY TO TEACH CHILDREN PATIENCE. OR, rather, to frame patience as "the art of anticipation" (Doesn't that sound so much more appealing and positive?). While everyone is waiting for dinner, you can talk about the meal you're going to have, show your child the dish, have them smell the aromas and savor the thought of eating a good meal. The French have a great saying for this: when they're feeling a little hungry close to mealtime and smell wonderful food, they say they are *mis en appétit* (which is perhaps best translated as "having one's appetite awakened").

I know this isn't easy. The "snack-time all the time" culture in North America puts pressures on parents to let their kids snack whenever they want, wherever they want. You're likely to encounter some resistance from your children (or their friends or other parents) when going cold turkey on random snacking. But remember: by scheduling (not forbidding) snacks, you're teaching your child important life lessons—and not just about food.

The Marshmallow Experiment

COULD SOMETHING AS SIMPLE AS FOOD CHOICES HELP CHILDREN DEVELOP important life skills? Yes! One of the most famous (and funny) experiments to demonstrate this is the Marshmallow Experiment. The results of this experiment show how food education is a means of teaching children good habits that will stand them in good stead for life: delayed gratification and self-regulation.

In the early 1970s, Stanford professor Walter Mischel conducted a seemingly simple experiment. One by one, the 4-year-old children whose parents had volunteered them for the experiment were invited into a small, empty room with only a chair and a desk on which had been placed a bell and a tray with two marshmallows. After each child was seated at the desk, the researcher made them an offer: either they could eat the marshmallow right away or they could have two marshmallows after waiting 15 minutes, while the researcher was out of the room. If they wanted the researcher to come back earlier, they could ring the bell—but then they wouldn't get the second marshmallow. Then the researcher left the room.

The hundreds of children who eventually participated in the Marshmallow Experiment were videotaped by researchers, who documented their behavior in detail. Some kids—the "low delayers"—simply popped the marshmallow into their mouths as soon as the researcher left the room. Others stared at the marshmallow for a few minutes and then rang the bell. One particularly savvy kid put the marshmallow in his mouth, but then didn't chew or swallow until time was up (although he drooled impressively). But some kids were able to wait, usually by distracting themselves: they sang, got up and walked or danced around the room, fiddled with the bell or chair, fidgeted, or even got under the table so the marshmallow was out of sight. At the end of 15 minutes, these "high delayers" got their reward.

Mischel's team followed these children as they grew up, doing periodic surveys and interviews. Their findings were astounding. Kids who were able to delay gratification (and wait for that second marshmallow) were more likely to be successful later in life. The "high delayers" were more likely to have better S.A.T. scores (on average 210 points higher) and go further in their education. The "low delayers" had, on average, a significantly higher body mass index and were more likely to have had problems with drugs. To some extent, these differences are innate, but Mischel also found that they related to family environment and parenting practices. Some kids didn't have the chance to practice delayed gratification as much as others. Those who did—for example, through saving up their allowance or not snacking in between meals—learned valuable life lessons that carried right through to adulthood.

Mischel also found that delayed gratification is something that most of us can learn. In later experiments, some kids were taught simple mental tricks (like pretending the marshmallow was a cloud) and were better at waiting as a result. This seems to be true in real life, too: a substantial set of kids who failed the marshmallow test went on to become successful, "high delaying" adults.

Creating an eating routine, in other words, is a great way to teach children some important life lessons. They'll be learning useful skills: moderation, self-control, and planning ahead. They'll also be learning to delay gratification and that you can make thoughtful (rather than impulsive) choices about eating. Scheduling snacks is one great way to teach these skills to children.

Creating a healthy snacking routine: Getting started

IF YOU'RE THINKING ABOUT CREATING (OR MODIFYING) YOUR FAMILY'S EATING routine to limit snacks, the most important thing to remember is that a routine will be positive for your child. This isn't about deprivation. It's about moderation.

You know your child best, of course. A set snacking routine won't work for some children with special needs. Children under the age of 5 (whose little tummies may need more frequent meals) may need a morning as well as afternoon snack. But the three meals plus one snack per day routine will work fine for most children 5 years of age and older. If snacking once a day is their routine, and if this routine is consistently followed, they'll adjust—probably faster than you'd believe.

You can also help your children wait longer between meals if you serve real food (rather than processed food) at both meal- and snack-time. In fact, the best way to think of snack-time is as a mini-meal. Try combinations of protein, starches, vegetables, and fruits, and avoid processed foods. Even "healthy" food pouches are to be avoided—they don't provide the same nutrients as real, fresh fruits and vegetables (and don't help much with table manners, either).

You can also use snack-time as a great, low-pressure occasion to encourage your child to eat real (whole, unprocessed) foods. Remember: if you serve a fruit and/or vegetable at every snack (as well as at every meal), your child will be much more likely to be eating their daily recommended amounts. Mealtimes will then be less of a battle. Snacks will work *for* you rather than *against* you.

Most important, choose highly nutritious foods for snacks. Wean your child off juice, which is mostly empty calories (apple juice has almost as much sugar as some soda brands, without much added nutritional value). Scientific studies show that children's interest in eating vegetables declines when they've had even a small amount of juice.

I know this isn't easy. Dr. Jennifer Cheng, who leads the Obesity Prevention Program at Harvard University, wrote about this in the *Journal of the American Medical Association*. When counseling a patient about her overweight toddler, Dr. Cheng suggested that water be substituted for juice at snack-time. The response? Her patient, Lisa, admitted that it was hard because her toddler, Maria, threw huge tantrums if she didn't get her way. Dr. Cheng showed them the Sugar Stacks website (sugarstacks.com) and asked Lisa to help Maria count the number of sugar cubes in a container of apple juice. Lisa's jaw dropped. "Wow, that's a lot of sugar!" Dr. Cheng worked with Lisa to develop new strategies (replacing juice with chilled water, for example). To help with the transition and give Maria a sense of control, she also suggested that Lisa ask Maria if she would prefer to have one or two small frozen juice cubes or a squeeze of fresh lemon or orange in her water. As Maria continued to whine, Lisa turned to Dr. Cheng and asked, "Is this what you call tough love?" Dr. Cheng smiled back and said, "I'd just call it love."

What to serve for a satisfying, healthy snack?

Healthy snacks combine foods that are high in nutrients and energy-dense. Grains (carbohydrates) provide energy for busy bodies. Fruits and veggies are high in vitamins. Proteins ideally also supply a bit of healthy fats, which helps with nutrient absorption and increases the feeling of fullness (satiety), enabling your child to last until mealtime without another snack attack. Pick one item from each category for a "complete" snack. Treat snacks as a mini-meal rather than serving snacking foods, but don't be afraid to make "fun" snacks, too, such as homemade popcorn with real butter.

Fruits and veggies	Grains	Proteins
Fresh fruit, sliced	Whole-wheat crackers	Nut butter
Sliced raw veggies (carrots, celery)	Toast	Cream cheese and/or dip for raw veggies
Fruit smoothie	Homemade popcorn with butter	Cheese
Vegetable (tomato) juice	Pita bread	Bean dip or hummus
Fruit compote (pages 263 and 277)	Low- or no-sugar breakfast cereal	Milk (2% or whole)
Stewed fruit	Muffin	Luncheon meat

New foods at snack-time: Fun games to play

THIS CHAPTER INCLUDES TWO GAMES THAT WILL HELP YOUR CHILD EXPLORE new tastes so they can expand their repertoire of snack foods. Grapefruit at snack-time? Why not?

Game 9: The Sour Fruit Game (Ages 2 and Up)

MAIN MESSAGE:

This game introduces your child to the idea that sour is an interesting (not necessarily bad) taste. Some of my test family kids went on to adopt grapefruit as their favorite fruit after playing this game. The point is to teach children to describe and understand the sour taste rather than just react to it. Older children will also learn that temperature changes how things taste. By playing this game, you'll encourage your child to like more "interesting" tastes so they can expand the range of foods they eat at snack-time.

My test families saw amazing results. Remember 3-year-old Lucas, who wouldn't eat a single vegetable before he started taste training? Lucas felt the same way about fruit. His mom, Jessica, told me, "Lucas would not even *lick* an orange." However, the Sour Fruit Game had a miraculous effect on Lucas. Despite her hesitations, Jessica began by telling him that they were going to play a "fruit game." Lucas loved the idea and was very excited to get started. With a little encouragement, he picked up half an orange and started licking it, imitating his mother: "MMMMmmm . . . juicy!" When Jessica told him it was sour, Lucas replied, "I *love* sour . . . This is my most favorite fruit, I think!" Soon they'd moved on to grapefruit, and fruit salad became a favorite dessert. Jessica proudly reported to me, "Lucas astonished his dad by identifying the grapefruit in the fruit salad, and proceeded to tell his father—who hadn't been there for the fruit game—all about grapefruit and how much he likes it. Success!"

WHAT YOU'LL NEED:

1 pink grapefruit, peel and pith removed, sliced
1 teaspoon granulated sugar
Fruit salad that includes grapefruit (at least ½ cup per child)

WHAT TO DO:

Taste test the grapefruit. Tell your child that you're going to play a fruit game, and that they'll have fun tasting different pieces of fruit. Give them two (small) pieces of grapefruit lightly sprinkled with sugar—one straight out of the fridge and one at room temperature—and ask them to taste each piece. Now repeat the experiment, but without sprinkling the grapefruit with sugar. Ask your child to compare the different tastes and sensations. They probably liked it better with the sugar and noticed the difference between the cold and warm versions. Ask your child to describe what "sour" actually tastes like. With some kids, this may work almost too well! One of my test family moms, Teresa, reported that her 2-year-old daughter was so excited by the discovery that she now calls grapefruit "sour" and asks for it by saying "I want sour!"

Taste test a fruit salad. Sometime later that day (or at most, a few days afterward), serve your child a fresh fruit salad that includes small pieces of grapefruit. I usually recommend using fruits your child likes (such as banana, apple, and grapes). Discuss the contrasts in taste with them and explain how combining sweet with sour fruits makes both tastier. Some young kids will find it funny to make the "sour face" after eating the grapefruit—that's okay. This allows them to express their reaction to sour tastes, but not to categorize that reaction as "ew" or "yuck."

Game 10: The Surprise Sack Game (Ages 3 and Up)

MAIN MESSAGE:

Our ideas about food depend on sight and smell as well as touch. If we can't see the food, our sense of touch can play tricks on us. This game helps kids refine their sense of touch and abilities to define textures, which is important for learning to like a broad range of foods.

In this game, a classic French taste-training technique is used to introduce an element of surprise into snack-time. It is used regularly in the French school system: kindergarteners play it in class, and teachers use it until the children are about 9 or 10 years old. Kids of all ages (and even adults) love this game because it is so surprisingly hard to guess correctly.

Safety Tip: If you're playing this game with a younger child, make sure the foods you use are ones you feel are safe for your toddler to eat, in case they do pop the foods in their mouth.

WHAT YOU'LL NEED:

A medium-size opaque bag (one you can't see through) with a smallish opening (a paper bag is ideal)

A variety of finger foods, including foods your child already eats as well as new foods

Note: You don't want the bag to be too full. I recommend including no more than one or two of the following: cherry tomatoes; grapes; olives; Cheerios, Shreddies, or Life Cereal; nuts (cashews, almonds, peanuts); raisins. Think of other fun combinations— use whatever you have on hand in the kitchen.

WHAT TO DO:

Hide the food items in the bag. Place your chosen food items inside the bag, *making sure your child doesn't see what you're including.*

Guess what's inside the bag. Ask your child to put their hands in the bag and to describe what they feel. Ask them to guess what is inside the bag. Then ask them to pick one thing and take it out. Repeat. (One of my test moms, Lori, reported that her kids guessed the olive correctly, but not the grape, despite being grape lovers!)

Variation: For older kids

Fill two dishwashing gloves (just the fingers) with items of different textures. Loosely close the top of each glove with an elastic so the child can't see inside but can wriggle their hand inside. Here are a few suggestions for contents:

- small rocks or gravel (smooth, hard, cold)
- baking soda or flour (dusty, dry)
- modeling clay (soft, squishy)
- a cut-up scrubby sponge (rough, abrasive)
- a cut-up soft sponge (smooth, squishy)
- a piece of soft fabric (silky, velvety, depending on what you use)
- popcorn, couscous, barley, lentils, or small seeds you might have on hand (smooth, hard)
- sand (granular)

Ask your child to reach inside each glove and describe what they feel. Ask them to use a variety of words (more or less complex, depending on their age) to describe the different textures. Have them investigate each item by pressing on the fingers of each glove and ask them to describe what they feel when they apply pressure.

After discussing the textures, ask your child to guess what is inside each finger of the glove.

The surprise sack game is akin to the many texture play games that preschools often use with children. Research suggests that younger children don't integrate visual and touch information in the same way that adults do, which is one of the reasons they can react so strongly to certain food textures. Research also shows that preferences for certain textures are learned, and strongly influenced by early exposure to a wide variety of textures.

Including food in your texture play is a great way to introduce young kids to the idea that foods have different textures. If they play with dried beans today, say, a slippery tomato or a bumpy cucumber will become less scary tomorrow. The possibilities here are endless: you can let your children touch and play with dried rice or dried beans (but watch for choking hazards), flour, sugar, even—although not for the faint of heart—Jell-O.

Top Tips for Healthy Snacking

- **Set a schedule** (such as three meals and one afternoon snack per day) and then firmly and clearly explain the difference between "eating times" and "non-eating times." Note: people's eating routines may vary, and you know your child best. Three meals and two snacks per day may work for some, whereas others will be happy with one snack. The important thing is to pick a routine and stick to it.

- **Do a snack purge.** Don't carry food in your purse or car glove compartment. It will be easier for kids to accept the new schedule if they know there's no food hiding in your pockets. Try to schedule your outings so that you're adhering to your schedule.

- **Be firm: don't let your child eat on demand.** If you're changing your routine, provide a simple explanation and then stick to it. Children may whine at first if you've been providing snacks on demand. If they see that you are firm, they *will* get used to it. They'll readjust their eating habits accordingly so that they're eating more at meals.

- **Make sure meals are filling as well as nutritious so kids eat well and feel less hungry between mealtimes.** Most people know that a balanced, varied diet is key to good nutrition. But one equally important (but often overlooked) point is that kids need a moderate amount of healthy fats in their diet for the proper absorption of many nutrients. A small amount of fat combined with other foods will also help kids feel full for longer (bread and almond butter rather than bread and jam; full-fat yogurt or cheese alongside whole-grain crackers). Incorporating healthy fats in meals increases the "satiety" (fullness) feeling and helps kids avoid grazing and random snacking between meals.

- **Treat your snacks like mini-meals.** Eat real, whole foods that you'd be comfortable serving at a meal (such as fruits, veggies, whole grains, and proteins). Healthy, filling snacks are best. Avoid offering standard snack foods, which are often high in calories but low in nutrition—those are "treats," not food. Teach your kids the difference.

- **Choose water or milk to drink.** Sweet drinks (such as juice, soda, or sports drinks) should be treats, not regulars at snack-time. Or try making smoothies with veggies and fruit (pages 251 and 267). Best of all, give your child some fruit and a glass of water.

- **Start young.** Create an eating routine that you'd like your kids to follow as adults. Unless you're dealing with specific medical issues, by the age of 5 (although in France this routine starts much earlier, by the age of 3 or 4 at the latest), children thrive on three meals and one snack per day.

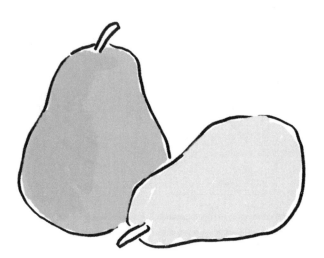

One Family, One Meal

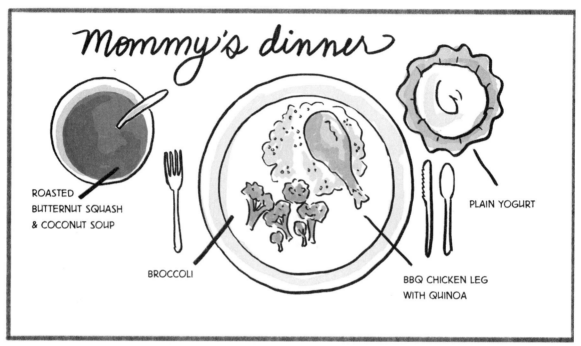

Mommy's dinner

ROASTED BUTTERNUT SQUASH & COCONUT SOUP

BROCCOLI

BBQ CHICKEN LEG WITH QUINOA

PLAIN YOGURT

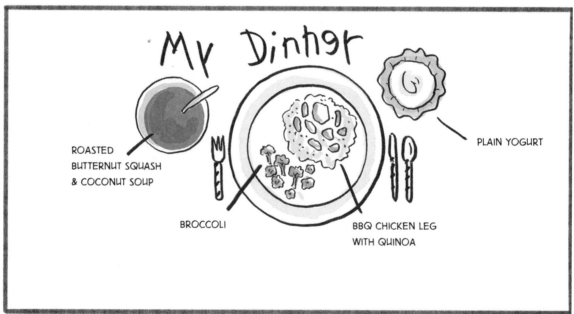

My Dinner

ROASTED BUTTERNUT SQUASH & COCONUT SOUP

BROCCOLI

BBQ CHICKEN LEG WITH QUINOA

PLAIN YOGURT

Routines and Rituals Make Healthy Eating Automatic (and Fun)

YOU KNOW THE OLD SAYING "YOU CAN LEAD A HORSE TO WATER, BUT you can't make it drink"? The horse (your child) has to *want* to eat healthy foods. But nutrition-based education isn't the best way to convince them to do so. Instead of focusing on nutrition, the easiest way for you to get your child to eat well is to create positive rituals for *when* and *how* they eat. If you create good eating routines and rituals, your child will be more receptive to learning to eat new things and to eating healthy foods, and they will truly want to do so.

Why are routines and rituals useful? To start with, they simplify your life as a parent. They create boundaries so that you don't have to rely so much on negotiating or imposing parental authority. For example, when your child asks for a snack 20 minutes before dinner, you can gently remind them of your routine (which might be something like "no snacks 1 hour before mealtime"). Good boundaries—for example, clearly separating "times when we eat" from "times when we don't eat"—mean less stress for you.

Good boundaries also create structure in your lives. This, in turn, provides children with a sense of predictability and security, and they won't be fussy if—in the run-up to mealtime—they're feeling a bit hungry. They'll also be less fussy about what they eat. If vegetables and fruit are served at every meal, and no substitutes are provided, they are more likely to eat healthy offerings as a matter of course.

Most important, these routines and rituals liberate you—as a parent and as an entire family—to focus on enjoying your food and on enjoying one another's company at mealtimes. Routines (which are best understood as good habits rather than strict rules) actually mean less work and more fun for you as a parent.

I know this sounds a little hard to believe, so I'll tell you a short story about two moms—best friends—who decided (after reading *French Kids Eat Everything*) to take a summer holiday together and turn it into a food experiment. During their holiday, the two families (with five kids under the age of 10) rented cabins together and shared the cooking. They set a schedule of three meals per day and one scheduled afternoon snack. They made simple, healthy, tasty dishes that the parents were happy to eat. One meal was served for everyone—no short-order cooking. If the kids didn't want to eat what was served, they didn't have to (although they had to taste it to see if they liked it or not), but no substitutes were provided. The parents decided they wouldn't nag, cajole, chide, or even comment. Their focus was having fun; after all, it was *their* vacation, too.

At first, it was nearly all-out rebellion. The older kids were unhappy and complained, and the younger ones followed suit. But the parents held firm. "It took about a week," one of the moms later told me. "But it really worked!" Once they realized that the new approach to eating was in place, the kids came to the table and ate what was in front of them. Less time as short-order cooks meant more time for the parents to relax. They were happier at the table—and their happiness was infectious. By the end of the week, the kids were eating on a schedule and trying whatever was put in front of them. They had tried—and, to their surprise, actually liked—a few new foods. Months later, their parents are happy to report that their children are still better eaters.

So what rituals work best? Every family is different, but this chapter summarizes some rituals that have been scientifically tested and proven to work.

The "veggies (or fruits) first" ritual

Does how we eat influence what we eat? I'd never really thought about this before having children. But after having children—and struggling to figure out how to teach them to become good eaters—I slowly realized that creating good eating routines is one of the most important jobs that parents have.

Perhaps the easiest yet most effective routine I've tried is the "veggies first" routine. *This sounds nice,* you might be thinking, *but my kids are not veggie lovers.* Well, if you adopt this approach, they just might surprise you. Researchers at the University of Pennsylvania studied the effects of serving a first course of carrots and found not only that children ate more carrots than usual, but also that they increased their vegetable consumption throughout the meal—eating more of other vegetables served later (including broccoli).

Intuitively, this makes sense. If you've adopted Secret 3 (no random snacking), then your child will be feeling appropriately hungry when they get to the table, and they'll be more likely to eat more of their veggies if those veggies are served first. Serving vegetables as a first course also makes eating vegetables automatic rather than a matter of negotiation. Because there's nothing else on the table (yet), your child won't be shuffling the veggies off to the side because something more appealing is also available, and you'll avoid the classic "No dessert if you don't eat your veggies" negotiation, which teaches kids that dinner is "yucky" and dessert is the reward. Instead, you're establishing a logical consequence: first this, then that. Until your child has finished (or at least tried) their veggie dish (Act One), the main course (Act Two) doesn't appear on the table. This is not a punishment, by the way, but rather a logical consequence. If you have a routine in place, your child knows that their veggie plate doesn't get cleared away, and the main course isn't served, until they've eaten (or at least tried) their veggies. This means that they'll eat more veggies—and remember, the USDA recommends that *half* of what we consume should be fruits and veggies.

Introducing a "veggies first" routine is harder, of course, if your child isn't a big fan of whatever is on their plate (cauliflower, anyone?). That's why teaching your child to enjoy veggies (using the taste-testing methods described in Secret 1) is the first place to start. Once your child has a set of veggies they like, these can start appearing in the first course. Try to avoid serving vegetables your child dislikes (or, rather, hasn't "learned" yet) as a first course. The test families I worked with while writing this book—many of whose kids disliked vegetables—all found that serving veggies first made a big difference. When he started his taste-training experiment, Jon's 10-year-old son wouldn't touch most vegetables. Brandy's 2½-year-old daughter wouldn't touch any fruit except blueberries (in blueberry yogurt, that is). By the end of our 3-month taste-training experiment, both were eating foods they had previously refused: Jon's son realized he loved green beans, and Brandy's daughter was eating fruit salad!

In another test family, Jessica (mom of 3-year-old Lucas) found that serving meals in courses had amazing results:

I've been doing "veggies first" with Lucas for the past few months. I love it! I think it's been the most effective way to get the kid to eat his veggies. I always start with a mixed green salad, cucumber salad, or carrot salad, or just toss some cut-up tomatoes and other raw vegetables in a vinaigrette. He seems to love it. I don't need to prompt him to begin eating now, which is huge! I'm embarrassed to say that prior to this, he ate no vegetables . . . zero. I could occasionally get him to eat a carrot stick with lunch. But now that he knows that his meals always go in a particular order, he's accepted it and digs right in. That's not to say that it was easy in the beginning. But it was amazing how little time it actually took before he began to ask, "What's my first course, Mama?"

—JESSICA

Joy, another parent, said this about trying a meal with a "veggies first" course:

We've switched to courses in our family of five (7-year-old daughter, 3-year-old daughter, 2-year-old son), and we've been skipping snacks, and they definitely eat a lot more vegetables. Serving the vegetables first, rather than American family–style of all on the table at once, has resulted in their eating more vegetables and less of the carbs/breads/pastas. I'm loving this, and the kids are enjoying it, too!

—JOY

If this still seems daunting, remember that kids are less likely to balk at smaller servings. Servings for kids are rarely larger than ½ cup, which is a lot smaller than a lot of people think (it's about four green beans or five cherry tomatoes). Servings are even smaller for toddlers: if your 2-year-old is eating 2 tablespoons of vegetables three to five times per day, they're doing well. By eating these smaller portions first, children appease their hunger, and they're more likely to have a reasonable serving of the main course when it does appear on the table. Automatic portion control!

The trick is to serve these smaller servings at every meal. Smaller kids need only about 2 cups (four servings) of fruits and vegetables per day—that would be a lot to eat for any one course or at any one meal. Instead, try providing one serving of vegetables as a first course at lunch, then one serving of fruit at snack-time, and then one serving of vegetables as a first course at dinner, followed by a fresh fruit dessert.

For older kids, you can progressively increase the serving sizes, as appropriate.

The most important thing about serving a meal in courses is that everyone eats the same thing—no substitutes and no short-order cooking. Kids do as we do rather than as we say; modeling good eating behaviors and healthy food preferences is one of the best way for parents to teach kids how to eat well. (The wonderful thing is that this structure will help you regulate *your* eating behavior, too.) Plus, think of how much time you'll save if you're currently short-order cooking for your kids.

The casual multi-course meal ritual

ONCE THE "VEGGIES FIRST" METHOD IS WORKING FOR YOU, WHY NOT introduce the multi-course meal as a family ritual? Unlike American-style dinners, in which all of the dishes are placed on the table at once, the French-style meal involves courses—as few as two courses (vegetables, then main dish) but more usually four courses (vegetables, main dish, salad and cheese, dessert). This strategy works wonders for encouraging children to eat healthy food: you separate the meal into different sections, and start with the foods you want your children to eat more of (like veggies).

Lest you think this sounds like a recipe for spending your life in the kitchen, you should know that on average the French spend only 18 minutes more per day cooking than Americans do. (Just as French women manage to look impossibly elegant while spending no more time getting ready than we would take to pull on our sweatpants. Annoying, I know.) Serving meals in courses doesn't mean spending hours preparing meals; rather, it means serving the different dishes you've prepared in a specific order.

You may be wondering, *When will my child be old enough to eat a multi-course meal?* It may be possible at a younger age than you would expect. By the time they're 5 or 6 years old, children can easily eat a three-course meal like adults, as long as the serving sizes are appropriate. Some start even younger. You know your child best—but remember, kids often surprise us with what they're willing and able to learn.

So, how do you serve a casual multi-course meal? It simply requires a little planning. Prior to inviting everyone to sit down to eat, place the things you'll need on the table: plates, cutlery, napkins, glasses, water jug, salt and pepper, a bowl of salad, a small plate of cheese, and any serving utensils required. A rule of thumb: you should only have to get up from the table two or three times during dinner. As much as possible, plan in advance for everything you'll need. Make setting the table a family event—kids love helping with this. Once the table is ready, everyone sits down to eat.

Veggie starter: *About 5 minutes.* Typically, a small bowl or plate is set in front of each person at the table, with either a small serving of veggies or—in the winter—a warm, tasty soup (such as Roasted Red Pepper and Tomato Soup, page 214). Once everyone has eaten their starter, the starter plates are cleared.

This doesn't need to be fancy. My mother-in-law sometimes simply slices an avocado in half, removes the pit, and fills the little hollowed-out space left behind with some home-made Classic Vinaigrette (page 302). The avocado (still in its skin) is eaten directly with a spoon. It's an elegant dish that takes about 30 seconds per person to prepare. *Voilà!*

Main dish: *About 10 to 15 minutes.* The main part of the meal usually consists of a protein, a starch, and a veggie side, served after the veggie starter is eaten. As the meal is casual, the pots or pans are often brought to the table and placed on trivets, and the food is served directly onto the plates so everyone can say how much (or little) they'd like.

On the weekend, when you have more time, a classic family meal might include Sweet and Sour Blueberry-Glazed Chicken (page 260), potatoes or rice, and a steamed vegetable such as green beans. Mid-week, or if you're in a rush, you might try making something simple in advance, like Ratatouille (page 217), which you can serve with couscous. The key is that everyone eats the same thing at the same time.

Salad: *About 5 minutes.* Salad is often a separate dinner for French (and Italian) families. You can serve it in separate bowls or on the same plate as the main course (unless the main course has a sauce or something else that would interfere with the taste of the salad). If you're truly doing this meal French style, you'll serve the salad with cheese, which will be on a small serving plate (people cut their own pieces). Usually one or two cheeses are served at most; everyone will take one small slice (about 1-inch square) to nibble with the salad. In many countries, such as France and Italy, people eat a salad course with most meals. This has a great effect on the kids: remember, multiple exposures to happy adults eating healthy foods increases kids' acceptance of those foods. According to one study, nearly 90 percent of French 8-year-olds like to eat lettuce. Eating salad is, for them, as normal as eating bread.

Dessert: *About 5 minutes.* Fruit is a good choice for dessert; this might be as simple as a pear, kiwi, or clementine. If you'd like something fancier, you can try adding a bit of ice cream or shaved dark chocolate, but the main focus of the dessert should be fruit. For the hot lunches prepared in French schools, the rule is fresh fruit for dessert 4 days per week, a sweet treat on the fifth.

This might sound like a lot of work, but my test families found that it doesn't take long to settle down into the new routine. Try it once per week to start with, and treat it as a bit of a special family occasion. To make it more special, use some of the fun dinner-table activities described later in this chapter. You'll find that your child will start looking forward to your meals together, and that these are great moments in which to introduce new foods.

The "polite no" ritual

WE'VE ALL SEEN IT: A CHILD WHO CRINGES AT THE SIGHT OF A PARTICULAR food, covers their mouth when the food is placed on the plate, and spits it out if it's placed in their mouth. (Actually, this is a pretty accurate description of how my older daughter used to behave as a toddler.) Teaching your child to negotiate a polite "no, thank you" is a delicate art—but one that will reap lifelong rewards. If children are offered a food, they're allowed to decline (after tasting it, if they're following the one-bite rule). If they don't like something, the polite thing to do is say nothing, but simply leave it discreetly on the side of their plate.

There's a practical reason to teach your child how to politely say "no, thank you": scientists have found that disgust is highly contagious. Children—even infants—are very sensitive to the food likes and dislikes of the adults around them. Basic rules of politeness about negative reactions to food will enable you to limit food dislikes spreading from one sibling to another.

Remember: refusing food is a great way to get attention—lots of it. The challenge for you is *not* to give your child attention for being picky. Give them attention when they're eating well. The behaviors you focus on are the ones that will grow.

Of course, parent-led modeling is powerful, but it can only go so far. Anyone with school-age children knows that peers have a powerful influence on children's food likes and dislikes. In fact, preschoolers are similar: even little children will be more likely to eat a food (or reject it) based on what other children are saying and doing.

One powerful experiment demonstrated peer influences on food preferences. British researchers decided to test the peer effect among young children. They created two "new" foods that the children (between the ages of 5 and 7) were unlikely to have experienced before: potato bread and quorn (an imitation meat), which were colored blue and given the names "fodrick" and "gwark." The new (and admittedly fearsome-sounding) foods were given to the children on paper plates, together with other snack foods (grapes, cheese, bread, and carrots).

The paper plates were presented to the children as part of a special activity day in which older children (8- to 11-year-olds from another school) were visiting the classroom. Unbeknownst to the younger children, these older peers were part of the experiment: they'd been trained by the researchers to encourage (or discourage) the younger children to eat the new foods. Praising the "fodrick" and "gwark" with lines rehearsed in advance, half of the older children ate the blue foods with gusto at snack-time. The preschoolers at their tables followed suit. The other half of the confederates refused to touch the food and made negative comments; children at their tables avoided the "gwark" and "fodrick" as if they were radioactive (and who could blame them)?

What's even more impressive is that the children who did try the blue foods were more likely to try other new foods in the weeks following the experiment—even without extra encouragement.

This suggests a simple ritual at mealtimes: inviting each child to say something positive about the meal. Negative comments can be kept to oneself; it's helpful to remind children that the polite thing to do when confronted with a food one doesn't like is to simply say nothing (or at least not to make a big deal of it). And, of course, it's important to respect the feelings and efforts of the person who made the meal.

You might even try some positive peer pressure of your own if you know a child (often older) who can act as a role model. If you don't have cousins or neighbors' kids handy, try to find a willing babysitter on your next night out. Instead of serving your kids pizza, try serving something adventurous that you know your babysitter likes. Or you might try finding an older child of a friend who might be a bit picky but would relish the opportunity to help positively influence your child. The older child might, in turn, be tempted to be more adventurous themselves—an unexpected benefit to his parents!

Online peers work well, too, such as the "Food Dudes" program (FoodDudes.co.uk), which offers rewards to kids who eat the Life Force foods (fruit and vegetables) favored by its superhero characters, battling with the evil Junk Punks, who are attempting to steal energy from children all over the world. (This cleverly uses "magical thinking": the qualities we associate with certain foods are often attached to the personality and character of those who consume them.)

The table talk ritual

AT OUR HOUSE, WE'VE RECENTLY STARTED ASKING EACH FAMILY MEMBER TO tell a story about the day. Cornell Professor Brian Wansink advocates keeping children at the table and taking the attention off the food (and power struggles at bay) through the use of distraction. Each member of the Wansink family answers four questions: What was the high point of the day? What was the low point? Whom did he or she most appreciate? What direction is your compass pointing tomorrow? (See Game 12: The Rose, Thorn, and Bud Game for a similar strategy.) It's okay to talk about the food, of course, but it shouldn't become the focal point of the meal. (Note: table talk is greatly aided by banning electronic devices of any kind at the table. This means you as well as your kids.)

Fun family conversations may have another unexpected benefit: getting kids to stay longer at the table. Make sure kids are comfortably seated; toddlers, for example, need foot support even after they outgrow a high chair. Try buying special kid-size cutlery for them, and asking them to set the table themselves. Tell jokes, tell stories, or simply chat. Parents are often at their most animated (and kids often enthralled) at the dinner table in countries where families prioritize mealtimes (think of every Italian family dinner you've ever seen in a movie). If you start telling some of your funniest or most interesting stories, your kids might surprise you with their sudden interest in being at the table.

"Happy meal" rituals

SPECIAL, CELEBRATORY MEALS ARE FOUND IN EVERY CULTURE. BIRTHS, deaths, religious celebrations, and historic events are all associated with special foods. Why not create your own meal rituals for special occasions? They create family great memories. Françoise, from one of my test families, sent in this anecdote:

> One of my best friends has a great family tradition. On each person's birthday every year they have a family meal (the friends celebrate another day). The kids decide on the full menu and then write it out. The parents prepare all their wished-for dishes. The only rules are that the menus have to be different every year and include a good variety of foods. So the kids really feel in control and creative. Also, they decorate the birthday girl's or boy's place setting with a crown of flowers and a little vase with a bouquet. And the

child or even adolescent sits at the head of the table! Now that her children are grown up (19 and 21), they all remember those times around the table as some of the best times of their childhood.

—FRANÇOISE

Other test families shared their experiences of creating everyday family food rules that made each meal special and more enjoyable. Here is a list of some of the rules I collected from my test families. Some of these were drafted by children, as you can tell! One last point: Too many rules all at once, or draconian enforcement, won't help your cause. The family table should be a place where you recharge your batteries and are positive with your kids, not a source of stress. Feel free to pick and choose the rules that might best suit your family, and remember: this list is aspirational.

- Wait to start eating until everyone has been served (my godmother calls this the "Royal Fork" rule—the kids love watching her, waiting to see when she raises her fork to her mouth, before they start to eat).
- Put the napkin in your lap and use it to wipe your mouth and fingertips (only). No crumpling.
- Every child should use cutlery according to his or her abilities (babies will be learning about spoons; toddlers about forks; school-age children about knives and forks, and which cutlery choices to make for different dishes).
- Comment nicely on the foods you like (and say nothing about the foods you don't like).
- Have a "nice eating face"—no noises, no slurping, no bites bigger than can fit in your mouth, chew with your mouth closed, the utensil goes in with a bite-size piece and comes out empty.
- Only polite requests for second helpings will be met (a logical consequence that keeps things positive but firmly polite).
- Adults must also be on their best behavior: no lectures and no complaining about the cooking or the food served.
- Children must wait until everyone has finished their main course before they can ask to be excused. (Younger children may ask to be excused when they are done, but once they are excused they can't come back to the table for more food.)

Some families write these rules down and stick them on the fridge as a reminder. If you make a list, involve your child from the outset—they'll take more ownership of these ideas if you do. Most important: don't get too hung up on policing perfect manners. Praising good behavior at the table will work better in the long run than commenting on bad behavior. The basic rules of politeness are meant to enable you to enjoy the meal together and to teach your child to be considerate of others at the table. Keep this goal your focus and keep your cool (no easy task, I know), and your child will eventually follow your routines. This might seem hard at first, but it will save you stress in the long term. As your child gets the hang of these new routines, they'll come to expect them—and even feel proud when they can help keep everyone on track.

Of course, whatever ritual you choose should be one that is fun for your family. Aim to make mealtime one of the most fun, relaxing moments that the family spends together. The two games below are designed to help you do just that.

Game 11: The Smiley Face Game (Ages 1 and Up)

MAIN MESSAGE:

This is one of the simplest games in this book and also one of the most effective. My test families were often amazed that even older children responded well to smiley faces on plates, in soups, and so on. Don't do this every day (or the effect wears off fast), but done once in a while, it is a great reminder that food can be fun. For younger kids, making a simple happy face part of their regular meal routine sets the right tone for eating healthy food in a fun atmosphere.

There are many variations on this game, but here's a simple example of a smiley face veggie plate that you can serve at snack-time or as the first course at dinnertime. Of course, you can invent your own options—or let the kids compose their smiley faces themselves.

WHAT YOU'LL NEED (PER SMILEY FACE):
3 or 4 cherry tomatoes
2 lettuce leaves
1 baby carrot
2 smallish cucumber slices

For the mouth: Cut the cherry tomatoes in half and lay them side by side in a semi-circle.

For the hair: Slice the lettuce into thin strips and mound it at the top of the plate.

For the nose: Slice the tip off the baby carrot (for a long nose!) or chop it in half and place it in the center of the face.

For the eyes: Use cucumber slices, cut as you like, and arrange them side by side.

Kids also love a "melting" smiley face as a garnish for soups and purées. Use little dabs of butter (or another soup or a garnish or purée of a contrasting color) to make eyes, nose, a mouth, and hair. Watch as your child eats up the smiley face—hurry up before it disappears!

Game 12: The Rose, Thorn, and Bud Game (Ages 5 and Up)

MAIN MESSAGE:

Family mealtime is a time for sharing stories about the day. Your kids will eat better (and find it easier to sit still for longer at the table) if you have interesting conversations to keep them entertained.

The Rose, Thorn, and Bud Game is one of our family favorites. Each person in the family takes a turn to tell everyone else about their day, answering three questions: "What was your rose?" (a good thing that happened today), "What was your thorn?" (a bad thing that happened), and "What is your rosebud?" (something they're looking forward to). This simple ritual avoids the conversational dead-end of "How was your day?" ("*Fine.*") and helps them appreciate that life is made up of good and bad moments—roses don't come without thorns, and there's always something to look forward to. Many families make the Rose, Thorn, and Bud Game a part of their daily dinner ritual.

Top Tips for Making Healthy Eating Automatic and Fun

- **Serve veggies first, at lunch, dinner, and snack-time.** You'll find that your child will automatically start eating and enjoying them more.
- **Use peer pressure positively.** Praise your child when they try something new or learn to like something new. Teach your child to *politely* say "no, thank you"—without criticizing the food—so that food refusals don't affect others at the table.

- **Use table talk to keep your child interested and motivated.** Ask questions and tell stories. They'll sit longer at the table and be more motivated to join you at mealtimes.
- **Use family food rules.** Rules will keep everyone on track and mealtimes happy rather than harried.
- **Adopt a motto.** "One family, one meal." (Or my personal favorite: "I offer two choices at mealtime. Take it, or leave it!")
- **Create special family meal traditions.** Whether once a week or once a year, your child will associate special meals with special family memories.

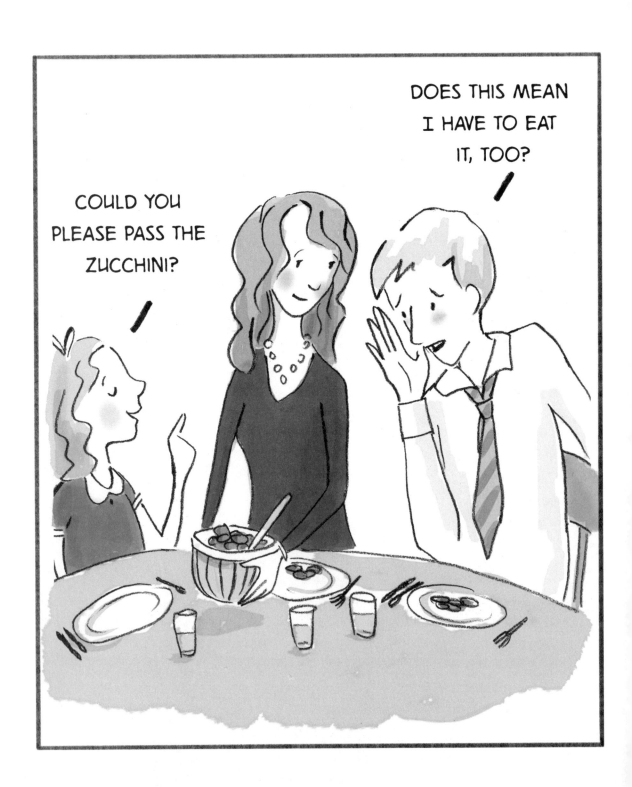

Kids Don't Need Kids' Food

IS VARIETY THE SPICE OF LIFE? THE JAPANESE (ONE OF THE LONGEST-lived, least-obese people on the planet) think so. Japanese tradition emphasizes the importance of a varied diet. Government guidelines advise both kids and adults to eat 30 different foods per day and 100 different foods per week! Children learn these magic numbers in nutrition classes at school. A traditional school lunch in Japan would include steamed rice with at least two fresh vegetables, fish, and fruits—a far cry from some of the classic North American standards (pizza for breakfast, anyone?).

One of the tragic ironies of the modern, industrialized food system (which is very good at distributing large quantities of food) is that the variety of foods we eat has declined despite the ever-increasing number of apparent choices available. Many kids eat a relatively small range of foods. For example, half of the vegetables consumed by children in the United States are potatoes—in the form of french fries. For many children, "kids' food" constitutes the bulk of their diet.

Is "kid-friendly" food addictive?

IS KIDS' FOOD A SORT OF "GATEWAY DRUG" TO AN OVER-RELIANCE ON PROCESSED food as a teen and adult? Sociologist and family food counselor Dr. Dina Rose thinks so. She argues that the high concentration of salt, sugar, and fat in many processed foods targeted at children makes them more likely to crave processed food as adults. These cravings may intensify over time. In a recent study of kids' ice-cream eating habits, researchers found that kids who regularly eat ice cream need to eat larger quantities to get the same sense of satisfaction (which was called a "high" in the ensuing media coverage). Former FDA commissioner David Kessler even argues that eating foods loaded with fat, salt, and sugar (particularly in the optimized combinations that the food industry uses) actually changes the chemistry of our brains, literally creating the conditions for addiction to fast food. Children, he argues, are particularly at risk: they have the most "plastic" (responsive) and thus vulnerable brain chemistries, and eating fast food young can literally hard-wire them to be fast food customers for life.

Dr. Rose summed it up best in her post on the *Psychology Today* website, where she argued that so-called "child-friendly" foods are addictive in the same way as drugs. She points to the fact that the vast majority of these foods are designed to give a flavor "hit" that unprocessed foods can't match. Kids get addicted to this flavor hit and come back for more. Once they're hooked, it's hard to wean them—as any parent who has tried to do so knows. Marketers know this, too: while traditional broccoli and corn producers are seeing slumps in sales, new genetically modified innovations such as Finest Supersweet Broccoli and Sunshine Sweet Corn are hitting the shelves, designed to cater to our growing habituation to sweet tastes.

Why is this a problem? Experts argue that giving mostly bland foods to babies tends to produce kids with limited taste preferences. As a result, some kids get "stuck" with a limited range of flavors and tend to prefer bland tastes and simple textures. For example, babies reared on white rice cereal are more likely to crave white bread.

Parents fall into the habit of feeding "kid-friendly" foods to their children for many reasons. We might assume that pickiness is a permanent part of our kids' personality, rather than a temporary phase, so we don't gently persist and help them get over it. Or we're busy, and it's just easier to serve the kids the same foods over and over again. Chances are that you know at least one child who doesn't eat any fruit or vegetables. Many more children subsist on a "beige food" diet consisting of white bread, pasta, crackers, and processed cereals (and I fully admit that this was my girls' diet when they were little, before our experiences in France opened my eyes). As discussed in Secret 2: Marketing Healthy Food to Your Kids Really Works, the result is a food literacy deficit: our children know less and less about food, and are willing to eat fewer and fewer things, raising the risk of micronutrient deficiencies, obesity, and associated health problems. This is an issue for families across the socioeconomic spectrum: under-nutrition (not enough food) remains a concern, even in wealthy countries, but malnutrition (not enough nutritious food) is also an issue.

It's not all bad news, though. Children who are exposed to more variety will have an easier time following a healthier diet; "taste training" has hard-wired their brains to be more receptive to doing so. This is true for adults as well: the Iowa Women's Health Study (designed to test the effects of healthy eating on breast cancer) found that women who started a healthy "real food" diet eventually developed aversions to the fast and processed foods they used to like. Kids *can* be weaned from "kids' food," as Jon, a dad in my test family group, found out:

> We had tried serving 8-year-old Sarah "real" chicken before, but she was always resistant. We used to take that to mean she was a born picky eater and would offer her something else for dinner. She loves breaded nuggets and used to have them two or three times a week. We used to buy big bags of them at the grocery store and keep them in the freezer, but don't do so any longer, so they are not an option for her. The other night, we made the Sweet and Sour Blueberry-Glazed Chicken [page 261], and I just served it up and mentioned how very sweet it was. Her 15-year-old brother didn't get a chance to say anything before Sarah scraped off the blueberries and quickly tried a small piece and commented that it was sweet. She then proceeded to finish that piece and ask for another, which she also ate. All without much discussion regarding the food! My wife and I gave each other the "don't say anything" look, as we didn't want to do anything to derail the success. Our son had a second helping, too. This was a first for Sarah—who had always refused to eat non-nugget chicken. It was a real breakthrough!
>
> —JON

Jon's story contains many lessons: if you serve food in appetizing ways, even the pickiest eaters may learn to like it; even young children can enjoy supposedly "adult" tastes; and perhaps the most important lesson of all, adults and kids should eat the same thing—mostly "real" food. Kids simply won't eat healthy foods unless you increase the supply of the healthy foods and reduce the availability of junk and fast food. The bonus is that eventually they'll start preferring (and even asking for) healthier foods. This has several advantages:

- **It's less work.** You'll be making one meal for the whole family (avoiding short-order cooking).
- **It's cheaper.** Do the math on homemade oatmeal versus those instant sachets and you'll see what I mean. If you don't believe me, visit the amazing "100 Days of Real Food" blog (100daysofrealfood.com), which tells the story of a family of four living on unprocessed, "real" foods for 100 days—all on a weekly budget of $125 (equivalent to the average family food stamp budget).
- **Your kids will eat better (and so will you).** Kids are natural mimics, and they'll copy what mom or dad does. If dad eats salad while sitting at the table, Fred will likely do the same. If dad gobbles cookies from the package while standing at the counter, guess what?

The wonderful secret weapon of this "real food" approach is the fact that kids' flavor preferences can also be trained to dislike fake food. Our daughters' friend Antoine—the son of French friends of ours who moved to Vancouver—is a good example. At the age of 3, Antoine refused to eat the store-bought, edible-oil-product-laced cakes served at the birthday parties of his new friends. "It doesn't taste good," was his response (and in my opinion, he was right). His mother proudly told me the story, affirmed by the fact that her at-home taste training had already enabled Antoine to detect—and dislike—the taste of mass-produced fake food.

Now, you may be wondering just what "real food" is. There are a million experts out there who will advise you on different diets, approaches, and gimmicks. I like Michael Pollan's definition: "Don't eat anything your grandmother wouldn't recognize as food." That means Go-Gurt is out, natural yogurt is in. Clif Bars are out, dried fruit is in. (There are more examples at the end of this chapter.)

A "real food" approach suggests that we limit the quantities of highly processed foods (such as sugar) that kids love. This is obviously important for our health, but it's also a question of taste. Lori, one of my test family moms, used this explanation with her kids:

> *I told our two girls that sugar is like a black crayon in a picture. A little can be really neat. But if you colored a beautiful picture and then colored over all of it with black, you couldn't see any of it. That's what sugar does to a dish: a little is neat. A lot hides all of the other flavors. Eat a lot of it all*

the time, and your tongue can't taste anything other than sugar. It makes for a super boring life. I love the fact that this explanation isn't about sugar being bad for you, but rather that it makes for a boring, monotone taste. It's so true. And I think that kids really understand these taste-based explanations.

—LORI

Weaning your family from kids' food: Do a family food inventory

AN INVENTORY IS A GREAT WAY TO GET STARTED ON REFORMING YOUR FAMily's eating habits. Start by making a list of the kids' food you have in your house. For each item, write down a "real food" equivalent. Hint: if you can't think of a real food equivalent, it's perhaps wise to think of crossing that item off your shopping list altogether. Next time you go shopping, try mostly buying from the real food category and limit the rest. It's important to limit, rather than forbid, kids' food, because you don't want this to backfire with a forbidden-fruit effect in which your child develops preferences for the very things they're denied. The best strategy is to divert your child's attention (by always having tasty fresh fruit on hand, for example), rather than appearing to police their eating habits.

I know that this sounds challenging. Think of it this way: in traditional food cultures there is no "kids' food." Kids eat what adults eat, and they do so at a young age; often as soon as they can chew or be reliably trusted to maneuver a spoon somewhere close to the vicinity of their mouths. Kids are hard-wired to be able to eat this way; they're more than capable of doing so.

When making your list of things to eat (and things to limit), remember: kids do as we do, rather than as we say. If you're eating lots of fruits and veggies, your children are more likely to as well. If you honestly enjoy them, you're increasing the chances they will as well. If you're trying new foods with enthusiasm, they're more likely to take a bite. Explaining why kids need to eat healthy foods helps (and certainly nutritional information can't hurt, in moderation), but most kids will learn best through consistent parental role modeling.

Sample Food Inventory

Kids' food item	Real food alternative
Sugary breakfast cereals	Slow-cook oatmeal (not instant)
White bread	Multigrain or whole-wheat bread
Yogurt tubes	Plain yogurt with a small amount of jam
Juice drinks	Homemade smoothies or lemonade (pages 251, 267, and 272)
Fruit leather	Fresh fruit
Frozen fish sticks	Fresh fish
Cheese strings	Cubes or slices of Cheddar cheese
Fish crackers	Breadsticks or plain buttered toast
Breakfast bars	Crunchy granola (try it with a bit of honey drizzled on top)

Weaning your child off kids' food will take time, but it's worth it. Essentially you're reverse-engineering the taste-training process, weaning your child from unhealthy to healthy tastes. Think of it like rehab for your child's taste buds! Once you have done your family food inventory and brought some new options into your pantry, there are three different approaches that you can mix-and-match: gradual substitution, the rotation rule, and the "try something new every day" rule.

Gradual substitution

ONCE YOU'VE DONE YOUR FAMILY FOOD INVENTORY, YOU CAN START GRADUALLY substituting real food items in your diet. Note: the following combinations are meant to allow you to transition your child toward healthier foods; over time, aim to reduce the processed ingredients.

- Switch from white bread to sourdough, and then to multigrain.

- Try making a half-and-half pasta sauce—half store-bought, half homemade. Over time, phase out the store-bought sauce.
- Mix whole-grain pasta with regular pasta, and whole-grain (brown) rice with white rice.
- Serve healthy breakfast cereals (for example, slow-cook oatmeal) and use the processed kind as a sort of topping.

We recently rotated through different kinds of oatmeal, convincing our kids that steel-cut oats were edible and then weaning them off the instant variety. Now they don't even ask for the instant kind any more. They had it recently at a friend's house and noticed it didn't seem as satisfying or tasty. Success!

Over the long term, your aim could be to transition your family to a healthier diet. Here are some specific substitution strategies that you might choose for your family.

- **Eat mostly 100 percent whole grains** (such as 100 percent whole-wheat bread, not white bread; ditto for cereals).
- **Make veggies and fruits half your diet.** Remember, half of our adult food consumption should be fruits and veggies, so your child should be working toward that goal. Serving veggies and fruits *first* at every meal is a simple way to help your child learn this proportion rule over time.
- **Eat healthy fats and avoid fake fats.** Don't consume high-fructose corn syrup (no sugary kids' cereals, no soft drinks, no fake icing—it's in a lot of stuff!) or anything made with hydrogenated oils or trans fats. Note: unprocessed fat (such as olive oil or butter) is not only okay in moderation, it's necessary. Kids need it for their development, and some vitamins are fat-soluble. Plus a little fat in a meal increases your feeling of fullness and helps you last longer between meals. This is one of the reasons that Harvard Medical School researchers have found that eating moderate amounts of healthy fats is a good strategy for losing weight and keeping it off.
- **Everything in moderation.** A little unprocessed fat, such as olive oil or butter, is okay. A little salt is okay. A little chocolate is okay. You get the point!
- **Teach your child the difference between *food* (which we eat often) and *treats* (which we eat once in a while).** At your meals, and at snack-time, eat food. Treats—including candy, cake, cookies, french fries, and cola—are once-in-

a-while treats. For example, we have potato chips at parties and whenever we have people over, but otherwise they're not in the house. This also helps avoid labeling foods "good" or "bad," which you shouldn't do, as it sets up emotional associations (like guilt) for your child and can lead to disordered eating.

- **Make sure your child gets enough water.** Juice is for special occasions. If your child wants to taste fruit, they should simply eat fruit.
- **Substitute homemade treats for junk food.** Good options include plain yogurt with a spoonful of fruit compote, juice and fruit popsicles, small amounts of good-quality chocolate, fresh and dried fruits, homemade popcorn, homemade cakes.

The rotation rule

NOW THAT YOUR CHILD IS STARTING TO EAT HEALTHY VERSIONS OF THEIR favorite foods, it's time to introduce a little more variety into their diet. This doesn't mean going overboard. Kids have their favorites (just like adults), and their individual taste preferences should be respected.

A degree of variety is, for most people, an ingrained habit. Many adults do tend to vary their meals. If you ate pasta for dinner last night, you're less likely to want it again the next night. However, it's easy to get into a rut of feeding your child the same thing over and over again if they accept very few foods. You can start to introduce variety by rotating your approach to making the dishes your child already likes to eat. For example, if your child likes cheese on pasta, serve shredded Cheddar one day and grated Parmesan the next. Or if they like raw carrots, try serving them cooked. Use the flavors they like to introduce them to new flavors (the friendly flavor technique discussed in Secret 1: Kids Can *Learn* to Love Healthy Foods). Your child is never too young to start getting more variety in their food.

More variety has psychological benefits: kids don't get stuck in liking foods or dishes prepared a specific way. They learn to expect novelty—and to enjoy it. My French sister-in-law even deliberately varied the heat of the formula in the bottles she gave to her babies so that they wouldn't get used to demanding it at one specific temperature. (Well, she did that deliberately with the first one, but it was a "that's life" parenting survival strategy by the time the second baby arrived.) You can also model this strategy for your child when you make everyday choices: "I had an apple at lunch, so I'll have an orange now." Variety makes things fun, and if food is less boring, kids will be more engaged.

The "try something new every day" rule

INTRODUCING SOMETHING NEW WORKS BEST AT A RELAXED FAMILY MEAL— preferably in the evenings, when you have time to talk about the food and aren't pressuring your child to eat because you have to run out the door. If you can't manage a sit-down family meal in the evenings, try leaving a little more time in the mornings for a more relaxed breakfast. Variety can appear at breakfast, too: you can serve different types of fruits, make new flavors of homemade smoothies, or serve different types of cereals.

The taste-testing strategies explored on page 32 will be helpful here, too, if you aren't already trying them. Remember: it's normal to have food preferences. We all do. Individual taste differences are real and to some degree innate. However, this doesn't mean that kids can't learn to like new foods. If you make a routine—one new food or taste every day (or week)—chances are your kids will be more cooperative.

Increasing variety: Keep it positive

WHEN INTRODUCED TO SOMETHING NEW, CHILDREN OFTEN RESPOND "NO" to the question "Do you like this food?" But how can they dislike it if they don't know it? What they really mean is that they're not *familiar* with it. It's your job to expose them to the new food, in as gentle and fun a manner as possible. (See the simple taste test ideas on page 32.) One of the best ways to help kids be eager about trying new dishes is to familiarize them first. Think of it as helping your child to get to know new people (each person has their own distinctive personality). Help your child warm up by introducing them to foods as if they were new and interesting characters in their lives. Let younger kids "meet" their veggies in raw form first. Toddlers can help wash them. Older kids can help cook them. Doing this regularly—and, for more selective eaters, *before* you ask them to eat these foods—helps kids get over their reluctance. Sometimes this means being creative about recipes, as Roberta, one of my test family moms, explains:

> If there's a food one of my kids doesn't like very much, such as eggplant, I try to serve it in different ways. This gives me a better chance of landing on a recipe that they actually like. Also, if they say "I don't like eggplant," then I can respond, "But you've never tasted it this way. I think this is the dish that will make eggplant your most favorite food!" This usually piques their curiosity, and they always try at least a few bites. Switching up cooking techniques also gets them to eat the food a few more times, so eventually

they simply get used to the flavor. I've seen this work beautifully with my 3-year-old, who now eats all the foods he "hated" 3 years ago, including eggplant. I started this process earlier with my other kids, so now even my 3- and 5-year-olds will eat bitter greens like arugula, radicchio, and dandelion greens with no fuss.

—ROBERTA

Think about what your child ate for lunch this week. In Japan (where children deftly handle chopsticks by the time they're in preschool), children eat fish and rice on a daily basis. In Peru, they eat quinoa porridge. In China, they might eat bok choy seasoned with hot peppers, or spicy noodle soup. In France, dishes like radish salad, roasted fish, and cauliflower casserole regularly show up on school lunch menus. As astounding as it may sound, kids actually *eat* this stuff. The reason is simple: they've learned to like it. In fact, they've been taught to like it—by parents and extended families, friends and peers, and teachers.

Some cultures are better at exposing their kids to vegetables than others, and at encouraging children to develop a broad set of food "likes." Chinese parents (and schools) have traditionally demanded a respectful attitude; adults disapprove of children expressing a preference for (or aversion to) individual dishes. In France, expressing dislike of any dish on the table is viewed as a serious breach of manners.

Remember: children increase their liking of vegetables, and their consumption of vegetables, if they are asked to taste them regularly (not just look, but *actually taste*). This effect is heightened if a greater variety of fruits and vegetables is present at home. This even works on babies: one study found that infants who were given a different vegetable every day for a week were more likely to eat yet another veggie—green beans, in this case—when it was offered.

French parents and schools typically adopt a "maximum variety" approach, and so French children have an expectation of novelty. Schools can't serve the same dish more than once per month. They even provide suggested dinner menus to parents to help them simplify the task of not repeating anything on that week's lunch menu. "We had chicken on Monday, so let's have fish today" would be a typical reflection from a parent. Contrast this with the North American approach, where the same foods—tasting exactly the same way—are served day in and day out. This increases the likelihood of kids having narrow, rigid food preferences.

Variety, naturally: (Re)Discover seasonal foods

A SIMPLE WAY TO MAXIMIZE VARIETY AND EXPOSURE TO NEW FOODS IS TO simply follow the seasons. With each season, new foods are available. This used to happen naturally: children got to know a variety of foods because they spent more time with adults preparing foods, as well as planting, cultivating, and harvesting them. My uncles and aunts, growing up in a large farming family, still talk about the fresh taste of the first ears of summer corn, the excitement when the year's first berries were ripe, and the flavor of home-grown tomatoes.

I don't want to romanticize this kind of life or minimize the backbreaking work that still goes with it in many parts of the world. My relatives also remember the sheer exhaustion of round-the-clock work in harvest season, worrying about the weather, and the missed opportunities as kids were pulled from school at a young age to help out on the farm. Nor was their diet especially diverse (an orange was a once-a-year treat at Christmas). But the fact remains that the modern food system—with its convenience and global reach—has broken the links between seasonality and family meals, and enabled us to cater to (and even foster) kids' limited food repertoires.

Think I'm exaggerating? A recent article in the journal *Appetite* shows that parents don't expose children to foods that the parents themselves don't like, which may make picky eating worse. Why? Because this will reduce acceptance of those foods in the long term, and negatively affect what scientists call "flavor learning." Researchers concluded, "To promote variety in children's diets, parents should model healthy behaviors by actively introducing new and previously disliked foods to their own and their child's diet, even if they themselves do not like these foods." The researchers picked vegetables that don't tend to be on the list of kids' favorites: Brussels sprouts, eggplant, and cabbage.

Read that list over again: Brussels sprouts. Eggplants. Cabbage. Do *you* like these vegetables? How did *you* react when you read them? Chances are you didn't like at least one of them. Now think of other vegetables you don't like. How many of those have you offered to your child?

My "vegetable I love to hate" was always cauliflower—I would never buy it, and was always surprised to see anyone eating it—but I figured out a cauliflower recipe I enjoy eating (Cauliflower Gratin, page 196). When my kids saw me learning to enjoy cauliflower, they followed suit. One child is more enthusiastic than the other, but both will eat it.

Our taste-training experiments have surprised even me sometimes. My 5-year-old daughter, Claire, is a good example of this. The other day she was dipping some veggies in homemade hummus with me. By accident, she got a small piece of raw garlic (I guess I hadn't quite blended it properly). "Ouch!" she cried, sticking out her tongue and spitting the little sliver of garlic on her plate, eyeing it suspiciously. "Drink some water," I said. But instead, she reached out and popped a piece of cut-up tomato in her mouth. My husband and I said nothing, as we know better than to comment too much when the kids undertake a food experiment. "It was stinging, but the tomato makes it taste better," she said, wonderingly. "I like spicy" was her conclusion. (Mexican kids apparently go through a similar process when they start to learn to eat hot sauce with every meal, at about the same age.)

Just to be clear: the goal of this book is not to get your child to enjoy raw garlic—I'm not even sure that Claire will be a garlic lover. The goal is to have children be open to trying new foods and appreciating food sensations—even apparently unpleasant ones.

Before you get started, remember the most important point about taste training: you need to believe that your kids *can* and *will* eat everything. Don't assume they won't like strong tastes or things that you don't like. Explore the tastes together as if you were on a fun family food adventure.

Fun games for introducing your child to more variety

USING THE THREE FUN GAMES BELOW, YOU CAN HELP EXPOSE YOUR CHILD TO variety in texture and color, and help them understand how "artificial" variety might be produced through food coloring. These games are particularly fun, as they all involve "fooling" your taste buds. (The recipes that start on page 175 are designed to foster a varied diet, as they present four different ways of eating common vegetables and fruits.)

Game 13: Terrific Textures (Ages 3 and Up)

MAIN MESSAGE:

Children often resist new foods because the foods feel strange in their mouths. This game introduces your child to a range of textures and enables them to develop a vocabulary for describing them. It will also help them learn to appreciate different "mouth sensations" without the pressure to eat that they might feel at the dinner table.

Make sure to do this experiment when your child is somewhat (but not too) hungry and explain that it is a "taste experiment" or a "fun tasting game." Make it fun!

WHAT YOU'LL NEED:

Choose two foods: one your child likes (the "I like it" food), and one they're learning to like (the "learning to like" food). The key is to vary the textures. For example, if your child likes apples, you would prepare (for each person participating in the game):

- 1 slice of fresh apple *(crunchy)*
- 1 small glass of apple juice *(juicy)*
- 1 dried apple slice *(chewy)* (you can make this by baking apple slices at 350°F for 30 minutes)
- 1 apple chip *(crispy)* (leave the dried apple slices in the oven for another 20 minutes, or until they totally dry out)
- 1 spoonful of applesauce *(soft)*
- 1 small piece of apple peel, preferably unwaxed and organic *(smooth)*

Do the same for the "learning to like" food. For example, if your child is learning to like tomatoes:

- 1 slice of unripe (green) tomato *(firm)*
- 1 slice of ripe tomato *(soft)*
- 1 small glass of tomato juice *(juicy)*
- 1 sun-dried tomato *(chewy)*
- 1 spoonful of tomato sauce *(soft)*

If your child doesn't like apples, try to think of another food that could be prepared with multiple textures. For some kids, this might mean using a soggy (soft) versus a dry (crunchy) Cheerio. Potatoes might also fit the bill (raw potato, potato chip, boiled potato, french fry). As long as it's a food your child likes that can be varied in texture, you can adapt it to this experiment.

WHAT TO DO:

Taste test the "I like it" food. One by one, taste each sample. Discuss which words you would use to describe each texture. Ask your child to describe other foods with similar textures, including ones that they don't like.

Describe the textures. Ask your child to identify the textures they like. Then ask them to identify textures they don't like (and encourage them to refer to these as "learning to like it" foods).

Taste test the "learning to like it" food. Follow the steps above: One by one, taste each sample. Discuss what words you would use to describe each texture. Ask your child to describe other foods with similar textures.

Describe the textures. Ask your child to describe the textures using as many words as they can. Make sure to try each sample yourself and comment on the different textures. In many cases, your child's natural curiosity will stimulate them to give the food a taste (or maybe just a lick at first). Be patient!

You can also use texture to add a bit of fun to your meals. For example, when my younger daughter (then a preschooler) was being picky about raw carrots, I bought a bag of baby carrots and cooked half (immersed in boiling water so they would stay bright orange), leaving the other half raw. I then put them on a plate on the table at snack-time, with a few cooked and raw carrots intermingled. I offered them to my husband as well as my older daughter. We had a great time guessing whether our carrots would make a loud crunch or be silent when bitten. After seeing us laughing for a few minutes with the "carrot crunch game," my younger daughter joined in. She delighted in making the loudest crunch of all!

Variation: Fooling Your Taste Buds

Older kids will have fun with this version of the Terrific Textures game.

WHAT YOU'LL NEED:
1 crunchy potato
1 crunchy apple
A blindfold

WHAT TO DO:
Prior to beginning the game, and *without your child watching*, peel and thinly slice the

potato and apple, making sure that your slices are as identical in size as possible. Cover them up, then invite your child to play the game.

First, have your child sit down and then blindfold them. Second, ask them to plug their nose tightly. Let them know they are going to get something to eat, and place a slice of either potato or apple in their hands.

Ask your child to bite into it and identify what it is. Then place the other slice into their hands, again asking them to taste and identify it. Ask "Was that the same food, or two different foods?" Most children will have difficulty distinguishing one from the other because the textures of apple and potato are similar and holding your nose makes flavors difficult to taste. Older kids will love to play this game on an unsuspecting adult.

Variation: Texture Play

A variation on this game involves texture play. If you have younger kids, you might want to start off with this approach. The main purpose of texture play is to give children a sensory experience about texture. Texture plays an important role in how food actually tastes and affects our perceptions about how filling a food is. Texture play gives children more confidence about different textures, and more ideas—and vocabulary—about the relationship between texture and taste. Here are some of my favorite items:

- baking soda and water (makes a gluey texture when squeezed)
- large dried beans (such as kidney beans)
- rice
- sand
- small dried beans or pulses (such as lentils)

Place each item in a separate cup and set the cups on a surface onto which your child can pour, stir, and manipulate the foods, then step back and let them play.

If your child is interested, you can also try manipulating the texture of foods with heat. For example, experiment with the texture (and taste and color) of peanut butter by heating or cooling it (or roasting it). Or allow ice cream to melt and then freeze it again.

Older kids might be interested in learning about additives that change the texture of foods, such as guar gum or xanthan gum. Next time you're at the supermarket, ask your child to read some labels for these additives.

Game 14: The Color Confusion Experiment (Ages 6 and Up)

MAIN MESSAGE:

This simple experiment teaches kids how color can influence their sense of taste (that's why processed foods often use artificial colors to increase visual appeal). This experiment also teaches your child to be wary of how their senses can be fooled through the use of artificial colors.

WHAT YOU'LL NEED:

5 identical drinking glasses (clear glass or plastic)
Water
5 tablespoons granulated sugar
Red food coloring

WHAT TO DO:

Prepare the experiment. Without your child being able to see what you're doing, pour ½ cup of water in each glass then add 1 tablespoon of sugar to each glass, mixing until dissolved. Now add red food coloring to each glass: 1 drop in the first glass, 2 drops in the second glass, 3 drops in the third glass, 4 drops in the fourth glass, and 5 drops in the fifth glass. The result should be a range of colors: from light pink to dark red. Each glass should look different; if not, add some more food coloring to the glasses as appropriate. Line up the glasses on a table. You're ready to start.

Observe the glasses. Invite your child to observe the glasses. Discuss the use of color in their everyday surroundings. What color is their bedroom, for example? What are their favorite colors? Then ask your child about the relationship between color and mood. Older kids may be familiar with the use of color by advertisers and companies (which know that we often implicitly associate certain colors with certain emotions). For example, green is supposed to be calming (think hospitals, waiting rooms). Red is supposed to be fiery and energetic. Blue is associated with grief. Ask your child whether they can think of emotions associated with colors.

Taste and rank the samples. Now, ask your child to taste the liquid in the glasses, *telling them that some are sweeter than others*. Ask them to sip each one, and have them rate the sweetness. Record the results on a piece of paper.

Fooled you! Reveal the answer: the five cups were equally sweet. Chances are, your child will have rated the darker drinks as sweeter in taste. Once you have revealed that they were all of equal sweetness, discuss the reasons they were fooled. Ask them about processed foods they might eat, or have seen other people eating, that use color to enhance taste.

Game 15: The Yogurt Game (Ages 6 and Up)

MAIN MESSAGE:
This simple game makes the point that our sense of taste can be fooled by color (and particularly artificial coloring).

WHAT YOU'LL NEED:
Vanilla yogurt
Yellow (or orange) food coloring
2 small bowls

WHAT TO DO:
Prepare the game. Without your child being able to see what you're doing, place an equal amount of vanilla yogurt in each bowl. To one bowl, add 1 or 2 drops of food coloring and mix well (the yogurt should have an appealing color and look distinctly different from the plain vanilla yogurt).

Taste test. Ask your child to taste the two bowls of yogurt and identify the flavors. Many kids will correctly identify the vanilla but incorrectly guess "apricot" or "orange" or "honey" for the other bowl.

Fooled you! After you've revealed the answer, ask your child why they thought that the colored yogurt had a different flavor. Ask them about the use of artificial colors in foods. What impact could this have on our experience of tasting those foods? Next time you're grocery shopping, have your child look at the labels on some of their favorite brands to see whether artificial colors have been used. They might be surprised: these additives are found in many common brands.

Older children may be interested in the difference between artificial colors (the most common ones include Red #40 and Yellow #5 and #6) and natural colors (from sources like beet juice, turmeric, and beta-carotene). You can also talk to your child about the relationship between artificial color additives and health. Some additives are proven or potential carcinogens. Some studies have also found a link between artificial colors and hyperactivity in children, leading the British Food Standards Agency to advise parents of children with ADHD to remove all sources of artificial color from their children's diets. The European Parliament passed a law in 2008 requiring products containing artificial food dyes to carry labels warning of the potential impact on children's behavior. The United States FDA launched its own inquiry in 2011, prompting some brands (including Frito-Lay and Kraft Dinner) to go "natural" and replace artificial coloring in its chips with natural coloring from a mix of beet juice, carrots, and purple cabbage.

Variation: The Soda Game

A fun variation to this experiment uses different colors of soda. Buy two or three sodas of distinctly different colors—such as cherry or lemon—as well as some plain, unflavored soda water. Prepare the soda in three cups, but add some orange food coloring to the plain soda. Then ask your child to taste it. Many kids will say that the orange drink (which is flavorless) tastes "orange."

Top Tips for Eating Real Food (Not Kids' Food)

- **Do a family food inventory.** This will help identify which "kids' food" items you'd like to wean your child from. Take the inventory list when you go shopping.
- **Use gradual substitution to replace kids' food with real foods.** Rather than going cold turkey, use this gentler method, which works well, particularly with older kids.
- **Pick a long-term "healthy food" goal.** Make it modest (one that you'll stick to).
- **Use the rotation rule.** Maximize the variety of the foods your child already likes.
- **Use the "try something new every day" rule.** Increase the variety in your child's diet. For more cautious eaters, try something new once per week.

- **Introduce your child to new foods before you serve them.** Kids can help pick, clean, and cook foods. Younger ones can simply look at the raw version before you work your kitchen magic!
- **Use seasonal foods as another variety booster.** This is an easy, fun way to make sure that you get maximum variety throughout the year.

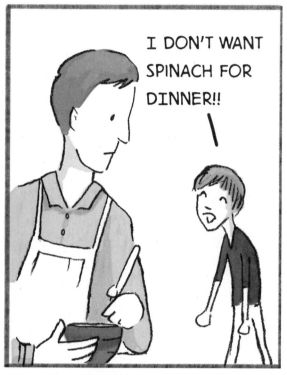

I DON'T WANT SPINACH FOR DINNER!!

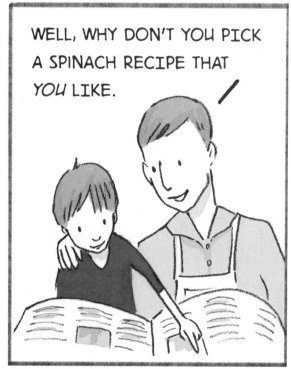

WELL, WHY DON'T YOU PICK A SPINACH RECIPE THAT *YOU* LIKE.

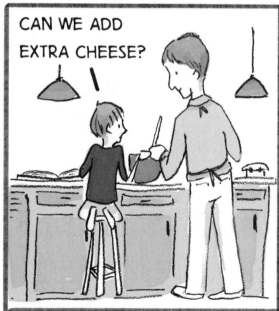

CAN WE ADD EXTRA CHEESE?

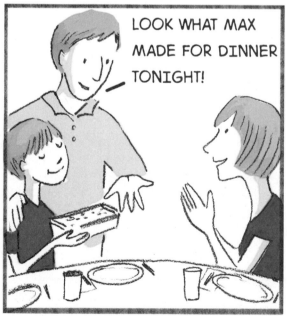

LOOK WHAT MAX MADE FOR DINNER TONIGHT!

Participation Works Better than Pressure

OW WELL WOULD YOUR SON PLAY FOOTBALL IF HE LEARNED ABOUT it by sitting in a classroom and watching a teacher talk about plays? Would your daughter learn to drive safely if she only watched videos telling her how important it was to "be safe"? Information is necessary, but certainly not enough. Our kids need to get out and practice until they have physically and mentally internalized the necessary skills.

The same is true with eating. Kids need to practice eating just as they would practice a sport (with you playing the role of coach). The more they follow their own interests and feel as if they are in control of their learning ("child-led," in parenting parlance), the more enthusiastic they are likely to be. Letting kids participate and take charge allows them to develop a sense of autonomy, mastery, and enjoyment that is key to lifelong healthy eating.

This chapter explains some simple, fun activities you can use to foster child-led learning about healthy eating. My test families experimented with these techniques with lots of success. The activities range from gardening to meal planning but share one goal: to encourage a child's involvement in eating, rather than controlling what the child is eating. This is based on the simple premise that kids are generally more eager to eat foods if they've been involved in their preparation, whether through picking, buying, preparing, cooking, or meal planning.

Too much parental control usually backfires at some point. In fact, it can have long-term negative consequences: parents who overtly control their children's eating behaviors (by preventing them from eating certain foods or saying things like "Stop eating, you've had enough now" or "Keep eating, you haven't had enough") are more likely to foster disordered eating patterns, like dieting or binging. Study after study proves that kids often show their independence by doing exactly the opposite of what we tell them to do. My favorite: in one experiment, parents were coached to prevent their children from eating an appealing-looking red snack food before leaving the room—after which most kids jumped on the candy and ate more of it than children whose parents had remained neutral.

Offer age-appropriate choices

One simple strategy is to allow children to make age-appropriate choices. For example, ask your toddler which vegetable side dish they'd like with dinner: carrots or green beans? Or ask your child what size serving they would like. Kids who are allowed to determine how much they eat develop a sense of their own hunger and also fullness cues, so they can start eating when hungry and stop eating when full. Serve small portions and allow them to ask for seconds (or even thirds!).

School-age children will appreciate having their feelings about new foods acknowledged. Although you may feel that you are offering encouragement, they may see your multiple attempts at "forcing" them to eat new foods as pressure. This is a delicate balance. Remember that although parents decide what, when, and how food is served, children should be allowed to decide *whether* and *how much* to eat—but they may only make that decision after tasting everything that is served.

Asking older children to craft menus is a great way to make them feel like their food preferences matter. French schools do this on a regular basis; the child whose menu is selected as the "featured" menu for the entire school feels seriously proud! You can easily do this at home.

Another strategy is to ask children to talk about eating behaviors (rather than nutrition) or marketing, to let them in on the reasons behind your family eating routines. Allowing children to buy the food (for example, selecting "their" beets to take home) and involving older children in preparing dishes (which adults should then enjoy with gusto) also often works wonders, as Roberta and Stacy, two moms in my test families, discovered:

Getting my three boys (ages 3, 5, and 7) involved in food shopping and prep is a big help. My kids love going to the grocery store and helping me pick out the fruits and vegetables. Often, I let them pick out a "funny fruit" to bring home and try. This is a really fun and exciting part of our shopping trip and a real treat for them. I let them search for a fruit or vegetable that we've never tried before (or rarely eat) that looks really funny or strange to them. They take pride in finding the oddest-looking one. Usually it ends up being an exotic tropical fruit (such as dragonfruit or prickly pear) and often they end up liking them. Sometimes they don't, but it doesn't matter all that much to it—it's the surprise of the experience that they really enjoy. Because they're the ones who choose the fruit, the experience is driven by them. This makes them eager to try it (never once have they turned down a taste of their "funny fruit," no matter how strange it looked on the inside). This has helped immensely in opening their minds and getting them to try new things.

—ROBERTA

Getting kids involved in the process is key. Last night I did a make-your-own salad. I put a big bowl of greens on the table along with small bowls of fruit (blueberries, mango, sliced green grapes, and dried cranberries), homemade croutons in star shapes, and salad dressing. (I purposely used fruit instead of veggies, thinking it would be less daunting to them; I also did the shaped croutons to make it fun.) Only one of my kids will eat salad normally. But last night, they came running up to the table and started serving themselves. Even my 7-year-old, who doesn't like blueberries and mangoes, started piling them onto his salad. I was blown away! Why didn't I think of this sooner?! But I am not complaining. The fact that they were willing to eat salad, and ate it so enthusiastically, thrilled me to death. My 4-year-old twins even asked to have it again tonight for dinner. But my husband was cooking and didn't want to do make-your-own salad. Instead, he just put salad on their plates: mixed greens with salad dressing, no fruit. My 7-year-old didn't touch it. The twins nibbled at a few leaves. But overall, I'd say this standard salad was a no-go.

—STACY

Of course, cooking itself can be a fun game for kids. Who doesn't like stirring the batter or squeezing juice out of fruit? You can try this at home or, if you're really lucky, find an organization that might be willing to provide cooking lessons at your school, such as Project CHEF, in Vancouver.

Get cooking!

Can you imagine a fourth-grade classroom full of kids happily eating kale and chard soup? Hard to picture, isn't it? But it's a reality in the classrooms that Project CHEF (Cooking Healthy Edible Food) visits in my hometown, Vancouver. The brainchild of Barb Finley (a chef and former teacher), Project CHEF works with public schools to provide hands-on education to primary school children. I recently had the pleasure of visiting a local classroom where Chef Barb was running one of her food education programs. What a treat! Barb and her team had transformed the classroom into an in-house cooking school, complete with a full-size cartoon mascot (a French chef).

When I arrived, kids were sitting at tables, each with its own cooking zone (a hot plate), prep area (including knives, graters, and other useful utensils), and a vegetable tray full of the raw ingredients that the students—each divided into teams of five kids plus a volunteer parent helper—were going to transform into a delicious meal.

Minestrone was featured on the menu the day I visited—but not just any minestrone. This soup featured fresh kale from the school garden, local herbs, and an amazing collection of vegetables from farmers' markets, including Swiss chard. *How is this going to go over?* I wondered.

Barb started the class with a discussion of the recipe ingredients, asking students a series of questions that had them raising their hands eagerly. "How many vegetables are in this soup?" had everyone counting intently. The answers (ranging from 8 to 17) had everyone laughing as Barb gently reminded kids how we define "vegetable": an edible plant (or part of an edible plant) without seeds—usually, the stem, root, or leaf of a plant. (This explains why tomatoes and avocadoes are technically fruits.)

The kids were even more attentive when Barb began making the soup, chopping the onion and then the other ingredients at her demo table, including some monstrous-looking carrots that had the kids gasping and laughing in appreciation.

"What's this one doing? The tango?" Barb asked, waving a gnarly, three-headed carrot at the class, followed by "We like vegetables with character, like this one. They have more flavor!" While Barb proceeded to chop and sample the "tango carrot" ("A good cook tastes her veggies!"), the class was utterly attentive: you could have heard a pin drop. When she slid the chopped onions into the olive oil, which sizzled away, the class reaction took even me by surprise.

"That's *so* cool!" shouted one boy.

"It smells *so* good!" said a girl at my table.

As Barb worked her way through the recipe, guided by the kids, they learned about everything from "measurement versus estimation" to the secret of cooking onions successfully. You could sense they were eager to act on Barb's tips.

"How do I cut this sage up?" she asked. "With my hands—a cook's best instrument!" Handing the sage to a couple of children, she encouraged them, "Now smell your hands!" Thirty pairs of hands reached for the sage leaves on each table, and I noticed the parent volunteers doing the same.

As the delicious smell of Barb's simmering demonstration soup filled the room, the table teams started to make their own soups. This went much more smoothly than I expected, as each child had an assigned role (which changed every day throughout the week-long cooking class): Cutting/Chopping, Supply, Washer, Drier, and Station "Meisters." Just like a line chef in a restaurant, each child had their responsibilities—a great way to avoid fights over who does what, and to encourage cooperation.

I admit that the chopping part of the class had me a bit worried. Thirty 8-year-olds wielding sharp knives? But I was reassured, as they had been trained by Barb and her team in "The Claw": a safe knife-handling technique. Sure enough, the kids folded their fingers back and hid their thumbs in a "claw" that safely held the veggies, while chopping everything from onions to garlic, carrots to tomatoes. Impressive!

Soon, seven soups were simmering away while the kids sat down to fill out worksheets. Barb took a few minutes to explain to me some of the secrets of the success of her cooking program. First, kids make a commitment on the first day: "Open mind, open mouth!" They promise to try everything, and the week's menu is designed to have them tasting new things every day.

Barb explained that positive peer pressure and the thrill of preparing foods themselves really help in encouraging the children to try new foods. She showed me the various lesson plans she had developed—all fully integrated with the educational curriculum. Interest has been so strong that Barb's classes now run 5 days a week, 9 months of the year. In some schools, her team will set up for a month, training the entire primary school in age-appropriate cooking skills. When Project CHEF leaves the school, teachers have new ideas about ways to incorporate food and cooking into subjects ranging from English and science to art and geography.

While Barb and I chatted, the children washed, dried, and stored their cooking implements (ready for use by the next class) and then set down to work on their learning logs, connecting the new learning to their lives. When they were finished, they began setting the tables with real china bowls and cutlery. Time to serve the soup! As it was lunchtime, everyone was feeling a little hungry. Meanwhile, curious faces peeked in the door (kids from other classes heading outside to play at lunchtime). You could tell by the looks on their faces that they would have liked to join us.

I sat down at a table with my own bowl and watched the kids around me. Many kids, Barb explained, didn't sit down and eat with their families. North American surveys suggest that 70 percent of families don't eat together on a regular basis. Kids eat at the computer, in front of the TV, or in their bedroom. Eating together, she emphasized, was one of the best ways to ensure kids accepted—and liked—healthy food. That seemed to be the case at my table. Three of the kids polished off their bowls and asked for more. Even the more hesitant eaters ate at least half their bowls. No one refused it outright. Looking around the room, this seemed to be pretty representative. Success!

While they were eating, the kids talked about their "table talk topic" (officially "autumn vegetables," although we did drift off pretty quickly into talking about video games—but at least everyone was chatting happily). Barb then stood to show the kids a package of instant soup and read out the ingredients ("Artificial color! What do they do? Put a crayon in there?"), before asking kids why making soup at home was a good thing to do. The kids had lots of great answers: It tastes better! It costs less! It's healthier! It's more fun! I can put what I like in it! It was clear that some positive lessons had been learned.

Clean-up was fast: the kids filed up and scraped leftovers into the compost bucket (which they would later take out to the school compost heap, next to the garden). Bowls were neatly piled, cutlery dunked in the big buckets of soapy water, and everyone headed out to play.

Like many local food education organizations, Project CHEF exists because of the devotion of a small team of dedicated people. But as Barb's team showed, it only takes a few to make a huge difference.

If you do try cooking with your child at home, here are a few helpful tips:

- **Pick the right time.** Ideally, choose a time when everyone is well rested and not too hungry.
- **Pick an appropriate dish.** For young kids, pick something simple. For kids new to cooking, start with something familiar so they identify cooking with something they already enjoy.
- **Don't worry about the mess.** In fact, kids are great at cleaning up—ask them to help. Toddlers especially love wiping, sweeping, and cleaning counters and floors.
- **Find "sous chefs."** Invite a friend or relative over or keep your babysitter for an extra hour. It'll be less stress for everyone (especially you) if there is someone else to help oversee and clean up.
- **Stay upbeat.** Praise your child for tasks they do well. If the recipe goes awry, just laugh it off. Remind them that we eat several times a day, and each time is an opportunity to start over and learn something new. Your child will learn a good lesson: you can learn from your mistakes, and "there's no use crying over spilled milk"—especially in the kitchen.
- **Keep it simple.** Small kids, basic tasks. For example, my younger daughter loves tossing the salad with vinaigrette right before dinner. This gets her involved in food prep and has definitely encouraged her to eat salad. A word of warning from experience: if you try this with your child, make sure it's a smaller amount of salad in an extra big bowl!

Project CHEF's classroom magic shows how powerful the simple act of cooking can be. Food is a sensual experience, and kids (even more than adults) are sensitive to physical impressions and sensations. Onions sizzling in a pan evoke an excited response from most kids—even those who might normally be indifferent or annoyed if an onion showed up in their soup. The simple act of handling vegetables helps "tame" them, making them less scary for kids. And kids are proud of what they create. Basically, children are much more willing to try a dish that they have a hand in creating—whether they're involved in choosing, smelling, touching, cutting, or cooking. (Babies, of course, can also play at cooking, even if this is limited to banging pots and pans with a wooden spoon to keep them busy.)

French families rely on this well-known fact to help kids conquer food dislikes. I've had many a proud French grandmother tell me about the personal food challenge she's orchestrated for her grandchildren. One was the mother of our friend Remi, in France, who explained her savvy strategy upon being told by her 9-year-old grandson that he didn't like zucchini. Her response? She went and bought several pounds of zucchini at the local market, and then she helped him plan a zucchini-based menu for a family meal (which included sliced zucchini salad as a veggie starter, zucchini quiche, and zucchini cake for dessert). The entire family enjoyed the zucchini and, despite his reluctance, her grandson admitted, "Maybe they aren't so bad after all."

One of my test families had a similarly inspiring experience. Lori's two daughters once held a long-standing aversion to "salad," a word they used to describe all green leafy vegetables. Lori, however, was determined to overcome their aversion to lettuce. She started by asking them to help prepare spinach salad one night, removing the stems and tearing the spinach leaves into bite-size pieces. To her surprise, they tore the leaves into much smaller pieces than Lori had been used to. Eureka! Lori also discovered that the kids didn't like salad with too much dressing. She began serving the dressing separately, and even asked the kids to help make homemade dressings with flavors they liked. This grew into a full-blown make-your-own salad game. Her family ended up creating their own "Kids' Salad" recipe (with mandarin oranges, toasted almonds, and even sliced radishes). I've adapted this idea for one of the games at the end of this chapter. *Merci*, Lori!

Get out your green thumb

ANOTHER TACTIC YOU SHOULD TRY, IF AT ALL POSSIBLE, IS GARDENING (OR the "green thumb gourmet program," as I call it). Gardening (whether at school or at home) helps kids in many ways: not only do they learn to recognize more fruits and vegetables, they're less likely to believe that vegetables taste bad—and so eat more veggies *and* a greater variety of veggies.

Researchers believe this is because kids are more familiar with the vegetables; repeated exposure reassures them and piques their curiosity. Note: gardening can be as simple as growing cherry tomatoes and lettuce in little pots on your windowsill so the kids can create their own salad. The research on the "green thumb" effect is so amazing that I've included more information on gardening on my website (**GettingToYum.com**).

Finding the balance: How much should kids decide?

THE OTHER NIGHT, WE SAT DOWN TO DINNER WITH OUR DAUGHTERS, WHO ate tomato-kale soup, followed by roast fish, potatoes, and one of our favorite carrot recipes, Vicious Carrots (page 190). We chatted and told stories about our day, and spent about 30 minutes at the table. Tempers never flared. My daughters (particularly Claire, who just turned 5) only required a couple of reminders to eat with their mouths closed and use their cutlery properly.

This sounds totally ordinary, right? When family mealtimes are working well, this *should* be totally ordinary—but all too often it's not. It certainly never used to be in our family. A few years ago (when our older daughter, Sophie, was 5), our mealtimes were often interrupted by tantrums about "yucky" food, constant requests for pasta and buttered toast, food refusals, and even walking away from the table. Mealtime was one of the most dreaded events of the day. My husband and I left the table feeling drained. The more we applied pressure—to sit at the table, to eat the foods that we offered, to use good table manners—the more our children resisted. We had created a bit of a battle-ground and weren't sure how to change the situation.

The secret to changing the situation seems counterintuitive: less pressure, less fuss. No coercion, and certainly no force. Relax. I know this seems like frustrating advice when your kids are jumping up from the table or putting napkins on their heads or calling each other names or gag-choking on the food that you insist they taste or when you're following them around the house cajoling them for "one more bite." But believe me, there is another way.

Think of your parental role here as one of coach. Observe and advise and help your child to learn eating skills. Don't take their food choices personally. Try to minimize or even avoid creating food fights; that way, food never becomes a power struggle but rather part of a routine, like brushing your teeth. Be nonchalant but cheerful about it. No coaxing, no hovering, no special routines or meals. Above all, if your child refuses to eat, take the food away without too much comment, but do not replace it with a requested favorite, no matter how hard that feels. They'll be hungrier at the next meal, which will work to your advantage.

Elizabeth Satter, one of America's best-known kids' food writers, terms this approach the "division of responsibility": parents are responsible for when kids eat and what is served; kids choose how much and whether they eat any particular item. The only thing I would add to Satter's approach is the idea that kids have to *taste* everything that is served, although they are not required to eat it. Of course, this approach raises the question of food likes and dislikes: How do we get children to actually *like* these foods? Repeated exposure (repeated practice) to vegetables is key, and this strategy is discussed in detail in Secret 2: Marketing Healthy Food to Your Kids Really Works (page 41).

There's another key role for parents: helping your kids develop the internal self-motivation to *want* healthy food. Your children should learn to eat healthy food because they *want* to, not because you *make* them. But the key to success is doing this in a low-pressure environment, which is the focus of the next chapter. Before that, here are some more fun games to foster your child's participation in building healthy eating habits.

Fun games for getting your child involved

FOR MANY KIDS, GAMES WON'T BE NECESSARY: THEY'LL BE HAVING ENOUGH fun helping you cook and bake. But the games listed below add an extra twist that will keep things interesting. And some of the games will be useful for reluctant kids. Game 16: The Mixing Game, for example, is designed to help kids who don't like eating combinations of foods of different textures.

Game 16: The Mixing Game (Ages 2 and Up)

MAIN MESSAGE:

What should you do if a child doesn't want to mix foods or let them touch on a plate? Put the child in charge. Even better: call it a game! This game will teach your child to enjoy different textures by allowing them to take charge of mixing food for themselves. It develops their "mixing" skills so they'll eat foods with combined textures more easily.

Note: The following steps should be carried out on consecutive days. If more than a week has gone by, you might want to go back a step.

Day 1: Mixing fun. Start with a simple mixing game that doesn't necessarily involve food you're going to eat. Provide your child with at least two bowls, each containing a separate ingredient. Some simple ideas for ingredients to use include two varieties of rice (brown rice and white rice); two colors of rice (you can use diluted food coloring on dry white rice—just be sure to let it dry); or two distinct types of dried beans (kidney beans and chickpeas). (Note: beware of a choking hazard with all types of dried beans.) Give your child a third bowl for mixing, a utensil for dipping and transferring, and a spoon for stirring. Then let your child mix away. As they do so, encourage them to notice how the mixing creates nice colors and interesting swirl effects. Encourage your child to touch the mixed ingredients with their hands. Ask them how it feels.

Day 2: Mixing a favorite dish. Prepare the ingredients for a dish your child normally likes. Show your child how you combine the ingredients to make the dish. If possible, have your child add the ingredients together and do the stirring. When it comes time to serve, remember to announce that this was a dish your child helped to mix. You may even want to ask your child if they would like to help with serving.

Day 3: Mixing at snack-time. Gradually introduce mixing at snack-time. Set the table with separate bowls of items your child normally likes. An easy option is plain yogurt with strawberry jam (or another flavor of jam they like). Place one spoon in each bowl and then provide your child with a third, empty bowl and another spoon. Ask your child to taste each ingredient separately, and then encourage them to mix up their own fruit yogurt to enjoy as a snack.

Day 4: A new twist on an old favorite. Prepare a dish that your child usually likes to eat. Choose one added ingredient that changes the dish somewhat, but not too much (such as adding ¼ teaspoon ground cinnamon to applesauce or 1 teaspoon dried parsley to macaroni and cheese). Ask your child to combine the ingredients themselves, stirring and serving as before.

Day 5: The "make it yourself mixed-up meal." Now that your child has some confidence in their new mixing skills, why not have a "mixed-up meal"? Choose a dish that's easy for a child to put together. For example, serve pita bread and place bowls on the table with ingredients your child likes to eat (whatever that might be—if it's blueberries and cream cheese, so be it). Allow them to stuff their own pita. They'll be much more likely to eat it if they're allowed to do it themselves.

Game 17: Make-Your-Own Kids' Salad (Ages 4 and Up)

MAIN MESSAGE:

Kids can learn to love salad if they're allowed to take control. Warning: this can result in some very strange salads!

WHAT YOU'LL NEED:

1 small head of lettuce

3 of your child's favorite fresh fruits or veggies

WHAT TO DO:

Explain to your child that they're going to get to create their own personalized kids' salad, just for them. Ask them to name three favorite fruits and vegetables. Next time you're shopping, bring your child along and ask them to pick out their choices. Once home, have your child help prepare the items (younger children can wash, older children can peel and chop). Have your child wash a few leaves of lettuce and tear the leaves into bite-size pieces to make the base of the salad. Then have your child layer their choice of fruits and vegetables on top. You'll get some weird and wonderful creations, but at least you'll be able to say your child likes salad!

Optional: Dressing is their choice, too. You might want to try my homemade Classic Vinaigrette (page 302).

Top Tips for Letting Your Kids Lead

- **Offer age-appropriate choices.** Giving kids completely free rein in the kitchen isn't usually a great idea, but allowing specific choices ("Would you like dried cranberries or blueberries as a fun topping for your salad?") gets kids motivated.
- **Get cooking.** Get your kids involved stirring, mixing, pouring, etc.—this works for kids of all ages. Older kids in particular will be more eager to eat the dishes they have prepared themselves.
- **Put reluctant eaters in charge.** If your child has a dislike for a particular food, they might benefit from a "cooking challenge": ask them to find a recipe that makes the food appetizing and serve it to the family.
- **Decide on your family's "division of responsibility."** Parents decide when the family eats and what is served; kids decide whether to eat and how much. This

works well for younger kids, but as kids get older, involving the kids more makes sense (older children may enjoy meal planning 1 day a week, for example).

- **Try gardening.** Growing, cultivating, and picking fruits and vegetables have a wonderful effect on many picky eaters. If you don't have a garden, consider visiting one or starting one at your kids' school or in the community. Farmers' markets are also great places to introduce kids to vegetables. Visit **localharvest.org** to find one near you.

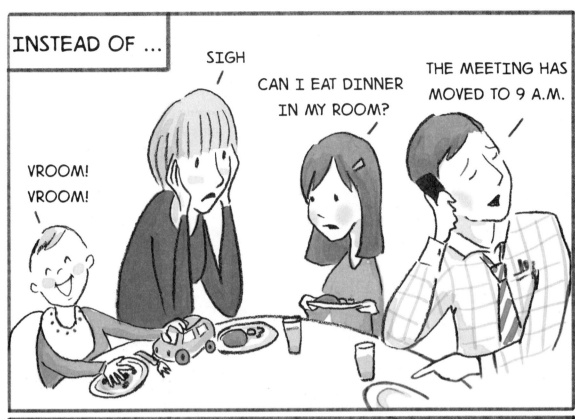

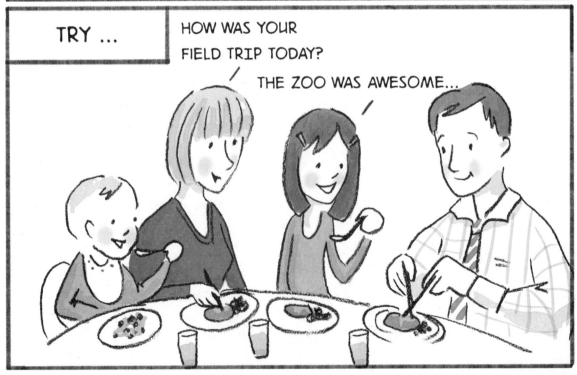

Secret 7

Mindful Eating Is Mealtime Magic

T HE "IG NOBEL" PRIZE (A SPOOF SPONSORED BY THE SCIENTIFIC humor magazine *Society for the Annals of Improbable Research*) is one of the most iconic—and ironic—prizes awarded to scientists. Brian Wansink, professor of marketing research at Cornell University and former prizewinner, certainly has produced research that, as the Society says, "makes people laugh and then think."

The experiment that won Wansink the prize was deceptively simple. He asked his (adult) research subjects to come into a classroom (set up as a restaurant) and enjoy a bowl of tomato soup. The participants—four to a table—chatted away, ate their soup, and then left the room when they were done eating. That, they thought, was that.

Except it wasn't that straightforward. Wansink called them back later to inform them how much they had eaten and to reveal the trick he'd used at the table: what participants didn't know was that two of the four bowls were attached to a tube beneath the table that slowly (very slowly) refilled the bowls. The people eating from these "bottomless bowls" ate 73 percent more soup than those eating from normal bowls, yet they didn't rate themselves as any fuller than those eating from normal bowls.

"This research shows that we eat with our eyes and not with our stomach," said Wansink. "The cues around us have a huge influence on not only what we eat, but also how much we eat and when we feel full."

Wansink, who has studied our eating behaviors for decades, has had much experience at proving to disbelieving audiences that overeating is often unconscious. As explored in his book *Mindless Eating: Why We Eat More than We Think*, we are prompted to overeat by everything from the size of packaging, plates, and containers to the names and labels of foods, lighting and colors, shapes and smells, and the organization of our cupboards. Kids serve themselves 74 percent more soda when using short, wide glasses, and people eat more ice cream when using bigger bowls.

But Wansink's work also shows us how we can turn this around: by being mindful of the choices we make. Simple strategies—such as using smaller plates and bowls, or reorganizing cupboards to hide junk foods at the back—can have impressive results for people trying to lose weight. Simply put: making poor-quality food choices more inconvenient is a great way to help people be healthier.

Certain trigger foods—simply by their presence in the cafeteria line or on the table—can encourage kids to consume more healthy fruits and veggies. In one experiment done by British researchers, placing a familiar fruit (like a banana) on the table next to a novel fruit (a guava) resulted in the children being more likely to try the new food. Changing the environment is also an important tactic, which is well understood by marketers and food companies. Mood lighting, bigger plates, supersize containers, attractive names—all encourage us to eat more. We can turn these tactics on their head, says Wansink, and make healthy eating "mindless" by developing daily routines and environments that promote eating the right amounts of healthy foods without thinking (or obsessing) about it. For example, serve new foods in very small containers (or even on a spoon) to make them less overwhelming in appearance for children. A simple placemat or tablecloth often works wonders, setting the stage for settling in at the table rather than eating on the run.

Many of these tactics are intended to "automate" healthy eating behaviors, just as Wansink suggests. As my test families found out (and as research verifies), these are useful tactics for improving your family's eating habits. But there's more to healthy eating than that.

From mindless to mindful eating

TASTE TRAINING ENCOURAGES YOUR CHILD TO GO ONE STEP FARTHER, BEYOND mindless eating to mindful eating. The phrase "mindful eating" might sound a little new agey, but bear with me for a moment. The slow and thoughtful eating championed by mindful eating advocates isn't really a Western rediscovery of Eastern philosophies. It's the rediscovery of something that our great-grandparents used to know—and that some (like the French) haven't yet forgotten.

Food is deeply sensual. When we eat a piece of food, our enjoyment is affected by our senses of smell, touch, sight, taste, and even hearing. Don't believe me? Try eating a piece of your favorite cake with your nose plugged or with earplugs in. Or try taking a bite and swallowing quickly, without chewing. You'll discover that eating slowly, using all of our senses, is the key to finding pleasure in food. In fact, the French have built their entire national school food curriculum around this insight: that engaging food with all of your senses makes you a more thoughtful—and thus better—eater. You'll be better attuned to your own sense of fullness (satiety). And you'll appreciate the subtle tastes of foods more (and not need the flavor hit of overly salty, sugary, fatty foods).

But eating is not purely physical, and it's not only about nutrition. It's also social and thus emotional. Pleasurable taste is important, but sharing food (or eating alone) also affects us emotionally. The difference between the preferred comfort foods of North American men (steak, pasta, burgers) and women (cookies, chocolate, and ice cream) is about *emotional* connections to food. As Brian Wansink observes, "Men prefer meal-related comfort foods because they make them feel special and well taken care of. Women, on the other hand, *don't* think of these as comfort foods. These foods reminded them of work—cooking and clean-up. Women much preferred the convenience of snack foods. Eating ice cream from the container equals no cooking and no clean-up."

How do we create positive associations with healthy food? The family meal is one of the best tools we have. All around the world, people celebrate formal gatherings—celebrations and festivities, christenings and funerals—by coming together to share meals. We do this because meals have the power to make us feel good—emotionally as well as physically. You know the wonderful, relaxed feeling you have after a celebratory family meal? Imagine if you felt that way every day! Not because of overeating, but because the busy world stopped for just a few minutes and you simply sat and enjoyed your food and the pleasure of being together with your family. This would have sounded unrealistic before I spent time in a country where family food culture is a priority: family meals, for the French, are akin to what Buddhists term a "practice." For the French, having a good meal is like going for a good run or getting a massage or doing a great yoga session. They feel relaxed, both emotionally and physically satisfied. The French even try to cultivate this in their children. Here is a quote from the Town Hall of Versailles (outside Paris) that describes their philosophy about school lunches:

Mealtime is a particularly important moment in a child's day. Our responsibility is to provide children with healthy, balanced meals; to develop their sense of taste; to help children, complementing what they learn at home, to make good food choices without being influenced by trends, media, and marketing; and to teach them the relationship between eating habits and health. But above all else, we aim to enable children to spend joyful, convivial moments together, to learn savoir-vivre *["the art of living"], to make time for communication, social exchange, and learning about society's rules—so that they can socialize and cultivate friendships.*

Food is (a little bit like) family therapy

FAMILIES, TOO, NEED TO SOCIALIZE AND CULTIVATE FRIENDSHIPS. FAMILIES need to spend joyful moments together, and to make time for communication and conversation. Eating is, in other words, a little bit like family therapy. Why does all of the research show that kids do better in a family that eats meals together, with positive rituals and routines? It's because eating is a way for families to negotiate togetherness, to reaffirm relationships. This is not always straightforward. It's about finding the right balance between love and limits. It's about doing your best and letting go of guilt when you (inevitably) make mistakes. It's about parents searching for their own personal "Zen of family eating": both an acceptance of where your kids are at, and supportive yet non-judgmental persistence with your teaching. It's about sensing when less is more: less pressure, less fuss, less rush, less choice, and (sometimes) less praise—being detached enough to act, rather than react. Most important, it's about love. Feeding is parenting: kids must have their emotional needs met (and have the right balance struck between "love and limits") to do a good job with eating.

Over years of cooking, I've begun to understand one basic principle: it's about "the love." My daughter always brings up the love in a recipe. She will look at a dish of sweet potato polenta with poached shrimp and demand, matter-of-factly, "Hey, Dad, did you remember the love?" In our house, "the love" isn't just some kind of sentimental way of saying we care about what we feed our kids. It is making sure the food is something they're going to want to eat. It's the skill of a chef who knows how to sell what he makes—how to market it, present it, and make it shine.

—JASON HAMMEL

Jason (a trained chef) intuitively knows what researchers have proven: if food is prepared with love and served in a warm, loving environment, children are much more likely to eat it. This is particularly the case when it comes to learning to eat new foods. If you find sources of pleasure and joy for kids in healthy food, it will become *their* comfort food.

I'm not saying that love will immediately solve all of your kid's eating problems! And I'm certainly not accusing you of not providing enough love at the table. It's simply a reminder: in addition to education and exposure to healthy foods, the most important ingredient of all is gentle encouragement. This is hard to remember when standing over a toddler with pursed lips at dinnertime, I know. But try to show the love you feel, particularly in those tough moments.

By mentioning love, I also don't mean that you should avoid conflict altogether (which leads some parents to short-order cook and let their kids eat whatever they want). Creating a healthy family food culture sometimes requires a bit of tough love to get to the point where you can be joyful at the table together. Industrial food culture presents families with new challenges that are very different from those previous generations have faced: an overabundance of high-calorie, low-nutrition foods, with no innate controls about how to respond in moderation (and in fact many pressures to do just the opposite). This is not just an issue in the wealthiest countries. Countries as far-flung as Brazil, Mexico, India, and China have similar problems. The good news: there's something you can do about it!

Of course, it probably won't be a quick fix. Creating a healthy family food culture takes time, requiring you to establish—and stick to—core values that may run counter to fast food culture. Doing so might give you some short-term pain, but the long-term gain will be worth it. You'll be giving your children the gift of the values and self-motivation to eat well—for life—by teaching them to be competent, autonomous eaters (without nagging, or bribes, rewards, or any other external incentives). These values will vary between families. For some, eating well is about personal health. For others, it might be about the environment. For others, it may be about spirituality, about treating the body as a temple or following time-honored religious precepts. Finding and sharing these core values with your children as they grow will be one of the best ways in which your family food culture becomes an enduring source of joy.

Tell funny jokes

You've probably heard (too many times) how family meals are the best preventive medicine for our kids. Children who eat with their families on a regular basis are less likely to be overweight or suffer from depression, and are more likely to do well in school. The challenge for many of us—including my family—is that life is simply really, really busy. If you have two working parents (our case) with no help at home (also our case), mealtimes are often a seriously stressful scramble at the end of the day.

To be frank, family mealtimes aren't always that much fun even if people have the time. Between siblings nit-picking at one another, complaints about what happened at school, stressed-out parents, and the all-too-usual comments on the food ("I don't like this!"), they can actually be a real downer.

So how can you put fun back into the family food equation? At our house, we've found that a little fun goes a long way. Of course, "fun" will mean different things to different people. Different approaches will work for kids of different ages. For some people, this may mean telling jokes (my test families had a lot of fun telling carrot jokes during the week they were testing carrot recipes). Other people might want to play simple games. Your goal is to create a light-hearted atmosphere of trust, acceptance, and engagement. I don't have to tell you that kids love jokes, especially ones that they can master and tell themselves. If family mealtimes have been tense, you can defuse them almost immediately by telling a joke—even if it's as silly as these. The jokes don't have to be brilliant. In fact, they can often be a little timeworn. They range from the obvious . . .

> *Q: What game do elephants love to play?*
> *A: Squash.*

> *Q: What sport do carrots play?*
> *A: Carrot-ee!*

to the subtle . . .

> *Q: Why did the carrot win a prize?*
> *A: Because he was out standing in his field.*

or even the risqué . . .

Q: Why did the tomato blush?

A: Because he saw the salad dressing.

Why slow = success

WHAT ARE THE ADVANTAGES OF EATING SLOWLY? IT ALLOWS MORE TIME FOR kids to describe their reactions to food (one of the most important elements in taste training). Rather than resigning yourself to "yuck" or "I don't like that," encourage your child to describe their sensations: "sour" or "slippery" or "rough." By talking about how food feels, kids learn to get over their first reactions to food, which are often feelings of caution or suspicion.

Eating slowly has another advantage: it allows the "fullness" signals produced by your stomach time to reach your brain (this takes somewhere around 20 minutes). It's a natural way to avoid overeating. Another great way to avoid overeating is to ask your children to gauge their fullness. Japanese tradition holds that it is best to stop eating when you are 80 percent full. French parents ask their children "Are you still hungry?" rather than "Are you full?"—a subtle but important distinction. It's an important lesson to teach your child, one that will help them naturally resist overly large portion sizes. (Portion sizes have increased hugely in recent years. In the mid-1970s, the average sugary beverage was about 13 ounces; today, it's closer to 20 ounces. Yikes!)

How many kids eat a hurried dinner in the car on the way to after-school activities, or gobble lunch at school before running outside to play? By doing this, our children are learning that food is fuel, that it doesn't matter what you eat as long as you fill up, that eating is an interruption in the day and a distraction from the productive, interesting, fun things in life. What a lesson! Consider weaning yourself off the "food is fuel" approach by committing to at least one slow family meal per week, even if it's a lazy weekend breakfast.

Changing your family eating habits will happen slowly, so you might as well enjoy the journey. Remember that although each change is incremental, they really add up. Our family is a good example. My two daughters are now good eaters, but they weren't always that way. In particular, my daughter Sophie, when she was 5, had a long list of "no go" foods when she was younger, including sandwiches, macaroni and cheese, and anything white and creamy (yes, even ice cream). Efforts to introduce these foods would be met with serious opposition, to put it mildly. Her younger sister, Claire, wasn't much better.

These days if you mention the word "Roquefort" to Claire she looks happy, as if someone had offered ice cream (and she *loves* ice cream). Taking a little morsel of cheese, she'll place it in her mouth and slowly savor it, clearly delighting in the salty, slightly tangy, creamy taste. The older and the moldier the cheese, the better. We once found weeks-old suspicious-looking leftover cheese in the fridge, glisteningly humid, with the delightful odor of long-forgotten wet socks. Undeterred, Claire delicately tested her serving and declared it "yummy," then requested seconds. I'm kind of amazed by this, but my French husband, mother-in-law, father-in-law, and our other French relatives and friends are supremely unimpressed. "She likes Roquefort? *Mais bien sur!*" they respond, with a shrug. "*C'est normal!*"

Most French kids love all kinds of dairy products; the French have, after all, invented more than 300 varieties of cheese. In fact, French kids even eat cheese every day at school lunch (rather than drink milk). In a nation of cheese lovers, one more Roquefort-loving kid is not going to get anyone's attention. When I try to explain to my French in-laws that I wouldn't eat anything except bright orange Cheddar cheese when growing up, and that knowingly selling moldy food (much less feeding it to children) could be considered a criminal offense where I come from, I get blank looks.

I now know Claire's penchant for the cheese is not miraculous. The reason my daughter loves Roquefort is simple: she was *taught* to love Roquefort. More precisely, she was given the skills to teach herself to love it. No one forced her. In fact, most parents know that force usually backfires. Even the youngest children can demonstrate a will of steel when confronted with a food they've decided will not pass their lips. Research suggests that forcing children to eat actually results in lower vegetable intakes, and a higher incidence of eating disorders, later on in life. In experiments, kids who are *less* pressured will eat *more*, and kids who are forced to eat may develop dislikes for those foods that can endure into adulthood.

Parents who are good role models are likely to have better success. Begin by asking yourself these questions: *Why* do you eat? What is the purpose of eating—for yourself, as well as for your children? Do you eat meals on the run? In the car? At the counter? How much is food a priority in your day? If food is a busy interruption, an after-thought, or a nuisance, your children will absorb that message.

Now consider this: What if you ate food slowly, savoring and talking about it, rather than rushing through the meal? What if meals (and, if you can swing it, a family meal) were one of the highlights of the day? What if preparing food together was something fun, a moment of connection, rather than a scramble at six o'clock, when you're fending off hungry kids from snacking while feeling stressed about the hassle of getting something on the table? What if trying new things was a shared family food adventure rather than a battle of wills?

All of this can be summed up in a simple formula:

Less pressure + less stress + more family fun at the table = more success

This formula assumes that picky eating is partly a power struggle. Of course, some kids have underlying health issues. For most kids, though, resistance to healthy food is psychological, not physiological. It might seem counterintuitive, but putting kids in charge of healthy eating, at an age-appropriate level, may defuse resistance and eliminate power struggles. That's the Zen of family eating—for kids of all ages.

Game 18: The Slow Food Experiment (Ages 6 and Up)

MAIN MESSAGE:
This game helps your child learn that the pace at which we eat our food influences how much we enjoy it. In general, the slower we eat, the better.

WHAT YOU'LL NEED:
A soft food that your child likes, such as cheesecake

WHAT TO DO:
Taste test eating quickly. Pick a calm moment during the day (snack-time or dessert after dinner) when there is nowhere to rush off to. Give a teaspoon of your chosen food to your child and ask them to swallow it without chewing. Ask them how it felt.

Taste test eating slowly. Ask your child to take another spoonful, this time chewing slowly. Ask them to compare the difference in taste during chewing and after swallowing. Most children discover that chewing actually releases flavor. Remind your child of the relationship between smell and taste. Ask, "How might chewing release smells that affect how you taste things?"

Chat about it. Talk to your child about times when they eat quickly. Ask why eating slowly may be a good thing for other reasons (social or safety-related). Ask whether your family might need reminders to eat slowly at certain times and what form these reminders might take. Younger kids may even enjoy having a secret code word or signal to use. For older children, you might want to explore the concept of mindful eating, as discussed earlier in this chapter.

Game 19: The Same Food Three Ways Experiment (Ages 4 and Up)

MAIN MESSAGE:

This is a wonderful experiment that one of the readers of *French Kids Eat Everything* designed to make variety fun for kids. (*Thanks, Stacy!*) It's a way to talk about food—where it comes from and all the different ways that it can be eaten. The idea is to provide one food in three different forms, to make variety fun and interesting for kids. In this example, spinach is used.

Note: Educators in the Slow Food movement use this idea for their taste-testing classes, too, but ask kids to try three types of apple, or three types of chocolate, and describe the appearance, tastes, textures, and aromas. You don't have to do this with spinach—pick anything you like.

Stacy, the mom who designed this experiment, had this to say about her experience:

> *A few days ago, I decided to try this game with spinach—one of the foods that my 4-year-old twins, Jamie and Reese, claim to not like. This time, I prepared a green smoothie with a large handful of spinach, a sliced banana, a couple spoonfuls of vanilla yogurt, whole milk, and crushed ice. Next, I sliced pieces of baguette and spread it with spinach walnut pesto (something that they like on pasta but which I've never tried serving on bread before). On each plate, I placed one fresh spinach leaf. I also added a second piece of baguette with real butter (I wanted to make sure that there was one item that they would be happy about).*
>
> *When I called the twins to come to the table for our experiment, Jamie was the first to arrive. He looked at his plate and said, "Oh, yummy!" (Not kidding!) Reese, who was trailing behind, sat down without saying anything positive or negative. I took it as a good sign. Jamie started by picking up the spinach leaf and asking, "What's this? Salad?" I said, "It's spinach." Then I explained that we were doing a food-tasting experiment. He proceeded to pop the spinach leaf in his mouth. Reese followed his lead. Next came the smoothies. They didn't say much as they sipped, but seemed*

happy. I then explained the gist of the lesson: I had served them spinach in three different ways—a plain leaf, puréed in pesto, and blended up in a drink. I said, "See how the smoothie is green? That's spinach!" Then I added, looking straight at Jamie, "You say you don't like spinach. But you do!" He said, "Yeah, you're right!" Finally, the baguette with the pesto. This was the one that I was most skeptical about. Even though they eat the pesto on pasta all the time, I wondered whether they would reject it this way. Nope—wrong again.

Every time that I've done "Food Three Ways," it's been a success. I think they like the "experiment" aspect of it, without any pressure to eat it. My kids don't always eat everything, but they almost always taste it without prodding.

—STACY

WHAT YOU'LL NEED:

Pick one of the fruits or vegetables from the recipe section of this book. Each fruit or vegetable has several recipe variations; pick two that you like. I recommend that you pick zucchini and make Melt-in-Your-Mouth Zucchini Purée and Roasted Zucchini with Cumin (both on page 239), reserving some zucchini to serve in thin, raw slices.

WHAT TO DO:

Pick a time when your children are not too tired and not too hungry, but still likely to be interested in food; snack-time is a good bet for most kids. Tell the kids you'll be doing an experiment, and invite them to the table. Have the three different versions of the food ready and invite the kids to try them in any order they like. Use the taste-testing ideas from Secret 1: Kids Can *Learn* to Love Healthy Foods (page 17) to encourage them to describe and then taste the food. Ask them to pick a favorite; usually even the most dubious kids will be tempted by this idea. Reluctant eaters will be encouraged if you try everything yourself. Remember: treat any refusals with as much nonchalance as you can muster.

Game 20: The Taste of Place Game (Ages 6 and Up)

MAIN MESSAGE:

This game introduces your child to the concept of *terroir*, a French word that roughly translates as "taste of place." Simply, terroir is the relationship between food culture, climate, and landscape: different places produce different types of foods. You can use examples from your region or well-known examples from elsewhere, such as maple syrup from Vermont, salmon from the Pacific Northwest, and corn from the Prairies.

Your children might be interested to learn that even the desert has its own terroir. In *Desert Terroir*, Gary Paul Nabhan writes about the ecology and culture of the American Southwest and talks about desert foods such as Mexican oregano and mesquite-flour tortillas. Rowan Jacobsen's *American Terroir* is another great book to read if you're interested in reading more about this topic. If you're scientifically minded, try researching (or asking your kids to research) the role that ethylene plays in fruit ripening, or climacteric versus non-climacteric fruits.

WHAT YOU'LL NEED:

1 or more ripe vegetables or fruits, preferably local (easiest if you do this in the summertime, when local foods are ripe for harvesting)

WHAT TO DO:

Introduce the concept of terroir using a simple explanation. Tell your child you're going to do a taste test of fruits or vegetables from nearby and far away.

Visit a market (optional). *If* you have a chance, take your child to a local garden or farmers' market to have them pick fruits or vegetables to use in this game and to talk to the farmers. Then head to the supermarket and buy the same fruits or vegetables from another region (chances are you may find one from another country). Good choices include tomatoes, peaches, plums, (podded) peas, beans, or peppers.

Taste test. Wash the two fruits or vegetables and peel or slice them as appropriate. Present them on separate plates (it's a good idea to use different-colored plates, so your child can tell which is which). Ask your child to sample them, comparing their color, texture, smell, and taste.

Chat about it. Talk about why the two fruits or vegetables are different. Older kids might be interested to learn that nutrients are higher in local foods that haven't been transported long distances or stored for long lengths of time. This means more freshness and flavor, as well as more nutrients and a lower environmental impact. Try following up by cooking a recipe that features only local ingredients. This is a fun summer project for kids—particularly if you put them in charge!

Top Tips for Zen Family Eating

- **Slow down.** The more slowly we eat, the better food tastes. In general, slower eating encourages more moderate consumption: the more slowly we eat, the less likely we are to overeat.
- **Lighten up.** Make it a routine to tell funny jokes at the table; a happier mood makes for better eaters.
- **Aim for mindful eating.** Use the techniques described in this chapter to encourage kids to be aware of the foods they eat; this will improve their vocabulary as well as their eating skills.
- **Grow your own food or seek out people who do.** Growing your own food is calming, inspiring, and rewarding for the whole family. School and community gardens, or your own backyard, are great places for the whole family. Plants in pots on the balcony (an herb garden, with tomatoes in the summer) are a fun, low-maintenance option.
- **Strike the right balance between love and limits.** Gentle, authoritative parenting at mealtimes will get the best results in the long run.
- **Treat mealtimes as family bonding time.** Kids are likelier to eat healthier meals if they have their emotional needs met. The family table is one of the best places to do this—in a low-pressure atmosphere.

Step-by-Step Strategies for Kids of All Ages

Babies: Feeding Maximum Variety with Minimum Fuss

It seems to be taken for granted in the United States that kids will innately dislike vegetables. But French mothers assume they will like them—and they do! I believe taste and appreciation of good and healthy foods, and curiosity for a wide variety of foods, can be learned and taught, and the earlier the better. Even my pediatrician was somewhat surprised that Pablo [18 months old] ate vegetables of all colors easily and thus didn't need to take a vitamin supplement.

—HÉLÈNE

WHEN HÉLÈNE GARCIA, A FRENCH-BORN MOM LIVING IN LOS Angeles, began feeding solid foods to her baby, Pablo, she did what comes naturally. She assumed he would be as interested in food as she was. Rather than treating it as a chore, she thought of feeding Pablo as a wonderful way for the two of them to bond and to simply have fun together.

She also knew one very important thing: the more you expose your baby to a range of flavors, textures, and tastes, the more likely your baby is to grow up enjoying a wide variety of healthy foods. Simply put, if you feed them white rice cereal, they're more likely to grow up liking white bread. But if, as Hélène did, you feed them leeks and watercress (at 6 months), and then salmon and kale purée (at 12 months), you'll have a baby who loves eating salmon-wrapped leeks *au gratin* (at 18 months)—as Pablo did.

The French don't have a monopoly on this approach, of course. Parents in many countries take a more adventurous approach to children's food than is found in countries like the US, Britain, or Canada. Mexican and Indian children eat spicy foods early on. Italian parents start their babies off with *brodo* (page 302), a delicious vegetable broth.

These parents know that introducing maximum variety (adapted to your baby's personal preferences and eating type—more on this below) with minimum fuss helps your kids get off to a great start. Luckily, most babies are naturally curious and treat food as one more way to explore the world. I know that introducing variety might seem daunting, but remember that the eating habits your baby learns in their first few years will shape their eating habits throughout life—affecting mental and physical health. What you teach your baby to eat will shape their preferences as a toddler, which in turn will affect what they are likely to eat as a preschooler, which shapes their palate as an adolescent and adult. Learning to like new foods isn't always a straightforward trajectory, but the effort you put in is—I promise—worth it.

Feeding your baby should be fun. It's a wonderful way to teach them about interacting with the world. Think of feeding your baby as a form of teaching—in which they're learning all sorts of fun new tastes, colors, and textures—the building blocks of their relationship with food. The more enthusiastic yet relaxed you are, the more smoothly this will happen.

Remember, by introducing lots of variety now, you're saving yourself time and stress later. The sooner your baby joins you at the table at mealtimes and starts eating baby versions (puréed, mashed, or chopped) of homemade, healthy adult food (without added salt and preservatives), the less work it will be for you. "One family, one meal" is a good motto to live by, and the recipes in this book will give you ideas of how you can take one vegetable and present it in age-appropriate ways for all members of your family.

When I launched an appeal for stories on my Facebook page, Catherine wrote to describe how she had approached food diversification for her two young sons. Working full-time with long workdays, she decided to cook during the weekends and freeze meals to be reheated during the week. When each boy was 6 months old, Catherine started cooking up purées with all of the vegetables she could find: green beans, cauliflower, carrots, zucchini, leeks, artichokes, broccoli, pumpkins, potatoes, sweet potatoes, even chicory. The purées contained a little potato and/or milk, so that the tastes of the veggies weren't too intense. Catherine did the same thing for fish purées so that her sons learned to like a wide range of fish early on. Her sons did go through the typical "no" phase at the age of 2, but Catherine held firm (not easy every day!), and the "no" phase ended—about 6 months after it started for one son and nearly a year later for her other son. By this time, Catherine happily wrote, they were "eating like adults." This doesn't mean that her children eat absolutely everything (yet). Now 13, one son still dislikes yogurt; his 10-year-old brother dislikes cheese and butter. But that's okay: Catherine encourages them and tells them they will eventually learn to like it. Catherine summed up her philosophy:

> *The point is that none of us would spontaneously choose zucchini instead of a good chocolate cake. But we can learn not to always choose the cake, and we can also learn to appreciate zucchini. Except if we've been taught that we can always choose the chocolate cake.*
>
> —CATHERINE

Luckily, as Catherine found out, your baby is on your side. Most babies will try almost any flavor you give them when they're young. They're naturally curious: just as they go for the new toy in the room, they'll go for the new color on the plate. That doesn't mean they'll eat it! You may have to introduce it several times before they accept it. Remember: variation is normal. What and how much your baby will want to eat will vary from day to day. Your baby's food likes and dislikes will also vary. Children will have a new favorite food that they may like for a week or two and then refuse to touch. My younger daughter, Claire, loved oatmeal for several months, wouldn't touch it for a few months after that, and then started devouring it again. Keep reoffering the foods from time and time, and they'll rotate back into your child's preferences again. This may have the added benefit of increasing your child's interest in food, as you'll be appealing to their natural love of novelty.

Which first foods should I start with?

THE MILLION-DOLLAR QUESTION FOR NEW PARENTS IS "WHAT FIRST FOODS should I give my baby?" Basically, science doesn't provide an answer. The most recent review by top American scientists simply notes that "there is no evidence for a benefit to introducing foods in any specific sequence or at any specific rate. However, it is generally recommended that first solid foods be single-ingredient foods and that they be started one at a time. The order of introduction of complementary foods is not critical.

Combination foods may be given to older infants after tolerance for the individual components has been established."

Translation? A mix of parental intuition and common sense is going to be your best guide. I'll explore some suggestions in this chapter, drawing on the French approach (as recommended by French pediatricians), because it emphasizes variety more than do that of many other food cultures. Note that I don't agree with everything that the French do. For example, despite all of the research demonstrating the advantages of breast-feeding, France has some of the lowest breast-feeding rates in the industrialized world, and if French mothers do breast-feed, they typically stop at 2 months. However, their approach to food diversification for babies is something that lots of parents around the world could learn from, and that's what I focus on here.

As you decide what to feed your baby, I'd also suggest drawing on your own cultural heritage combined with common sense (and discussions with your health-care provider as appropriate). Dr. Jatinder Bhatia (Chief Neonatologist at Georgia Health Science University and member of the American Academy of Pediatrics Committee on Nutrition) argues that Canadian and American guidelines contain a cultural bias that fails to reflect our ethnic diversity. He recommends feeding mild curries to babies!

You might be happy to know that your baby has been learning about flavors since even before starting solid foods—and even before birth. Foods eaten by women during pregnancy flavor the amniotic fluid and thus influence babies' taste preferences.If you eat lots of strong-flavored greens (such as arugula) during your pregnancy, chances are that your child will love these, too. (I realize now that my love of grilled cheese sandwiches—one of the only things I could eat during my first pregnancy without throwing up—was probably not the best tactic for raising a happy omnivore!)

What you eat also flavors your breast milk, so babies continue to encounter new flavors early on. Some studies have even found that varying the flavor of formula (for bottle-fed babies) can also increase the acceptance of specific foods later on. What does this mean? Simply put, although we are born with certain preferences, our experiences are profoundly important in shaping what we like to eat. The best time in a child's life to shape their food preferences is before the age of 2, when most children hit the "no" stage and many also develop temporary neophobia (fear of new foods). Knowing this, French parents (like many parents around the world) aim to develop their baby's love of a wide range of foods between 6 and 24 months of age.

The French even have a phrase for this: *l'éducation du goût* (the education of taste). And they speak rather poetically about the "*debut de la diversification*" (beginning of food diversification), with the same emotion that parents in many cultures reserve for the moment when their child starts school or takes their first step. When a child starts eating solid foods, they're starting a long and interesting journey. Quite the contrast to the dull, prosaic English equivalent: "starting solid foods."

How does early food diversification work, practically speaking? Take the case of Hélène, the French mom living in LA and blogging at frenchfoodiebaby.blogspot.ca. When she started her son, Pablo, on solid foods, she started with vegetable purées. Why veggies first? Delaying fruit for at least a month, so babies get used to the less-sweet taste of vegetables, is a standard recommendation of French pediatricians. Not all French parents follow this rule, but it seems to make sense to include as many veggies as fruits in your baby's menu. Hélène introduced the following vegetables, one after the other, waiting 2 or 3 days between each to see if Pablo had any signs of allergic reactions (he didn't). By the age of 8 months, here's what Pablo was eating:

- **Asparagus** (green), steamed with a bit of potato and puréed
- **Beans** (green), steamed and puréed
- **Broccoli**, steamed and puréed
- **Brussels sprouts**, boiled (not steamed, so they're less bitter) with a bit of potato and puréed
- **Carrots**, steamed and puréed
- **Cauliflower**, steamed and puréed
- **Celery root**, steamed with a bit of potato and puréed
- **Cucumber**, steamed with a bit of potato and puréed
- **Endive**, steamed with a bit of potato and puréed
- **Kale/all chards**, steamed with a bit of potato and puréed
- **Peas**, steamed and puréed
- **Sweet potato**, steamed and puréed
- **Watercress**, steamed with a bit of potato and puréed
- **White leeks**, steamed with a bit of potato and puréed (only the top white part of the leek)
- **Winter squash**, steamed and puréed
- **Zucchini**, steamed with a bit of potato and puréed

This is quite the list. But it's not out of the ordinary for French parents. In practice, French parents introduce a new vegetable every few days. A recent study found that they introduced, on average, 6 new veggies in the first month of solid foods, and nearly half the babies in the study were introduced to between 7 and 12 veggies in the first month. French mothers also rotated vegetables on a daily and weekly basis: they made, on average, 18 changes to the way they prepared the vegetables they offered (some made as many as 27 changes!). The result? French babies are eating—and enjoying—a much greater variety of foods by the time they're 2 years old—just when the picky eating phase hits. By the time they are school-age, most have got over the picky eating phase. Of course, they're still learning to like a broader variety of foods, but few are on the "beige food" diet that's common in North America.

The list of "first food" vegetables recommended by the French Society of Pediatrics (FSP) might surprise a lot of American parents. According to their official baby-feeding guide, babies as young as 5 or 6 months can be introduced to all of the following (in any order) as smooth purées, any of which can be mixed into a small amount of potatoes, which should be introduced separately first, just as Hélène did: carrots, green beans, spinach, zucchini (peeled and seeds removed), leeks (whites only), pumpkin, baby endive and baby chard (in limited quantities), and green peas only if they are "extra-fine" and served in small quantities (the French think that green peas are really hard on the digestive system and don't tend to serve them until the babies are a bit older). French pediatricians think these veggies are easy to digest and suitable from 6 months onward.

If you think that sounds impressive, you'll be even more impressed by the foods the FSP recommends introducing from 9 months onward: cabbage, turnip, onion, leek (white part only), celery, celery root (celeriac), green peas, tomatoes, Jerusalem artichoke (sunchokes), cardoons, artichoke, peppers, eggplant, and parsley. If these are handled well, then it's on to others, including fennel, cauliflower, broccoli, and beets. (Hélène appears to have jumped the gun on some of these.) Any of these vegetables can now be combined with fish. Indeed, 9-month-old Pablo was eating purée combinations ranging from sole and cucumber to salmon and sorrel to cod and chard! The purées at this age are slightly thicker, or may have small lumps or be combined with small pieces of pasta (such as orzo).

Once meat options are introduced, the meals become even more interesting. By the time he was a year old, Pablo was eating chicken *jardinière* (with carrot, turnip, green beans, and flat-leaf parsley), veal and green asparagus (tips only), and (my personal favorite) lamb and rutabaga purée (by this time a lumpier dish with small, chewable morsels). Pablo had also transitioned to finger foods.

Here's one of Pablo's sample daily menus from when he was 13 months old. Note: both lunch and dinner follow the traditional four-course meal structure: appetizer, main course, cheese course, dessert.

BREAKFAST
Baby oatmeal with milk
Fruit (berries)
Plain Greek yogurt with a sprinkle of wheat germ
Orange juice

LUNCH
Appetizer/finger foods: Greek salad (grated cucumber, tomatoes, feta cheese)
Main course: *Boeuf ratatouille* purée
Cheese: Gouda
Dessert: Yogurt and fresh apricot slices

SNACK
Apple-pear compote

DINNER
Appetizer/finger foods: Endive and green bean salad with blue cheese
Main course: Roasted pork ribs (small pieces from his parents' servings), herbed broccoli purée
Cheese: Petit Basque sheep's milk cheese
Dessert: Plain Greek yogurt

On his 18-month "birthday," Pablo's lunch menu looked like this:

- *Appetizer/finger foods*: Cold (cooked) zucchini, mint, and feta salad
- *Main course*: Veal liver with green beans (with garlic and flat-leaf parsley)
- *Cheese:* Creamy Italian blue cheese
- *Dessert:* Plain yogurt with fresh fruit

For his afternoon snack, Pablo ate persimmon seeds; dinner included roasted butternut squash and coconut soup, Dover sole fillets with quinoa, and Camembert! Hélène explains that Pablo is simply eating what the adults are eating, appropriately adapted (for example, his fish is cut up carefully to make sure there are no bones). Indeed, the FSP suggests that babies from 18 months onward can eat nearly everything adults eat (although it recommends waiting on dried beans such as kidney beans until they can chew them properly, otherwise they present a choking hazard).

When *New York Times* reporter Keith Dixon tried this with his 8-month-old daughter, Gracie, he was pleasantly surprised by the results. With the help of a food mill, little Gracie happily devoured ravioli with sage butter, pecorino, and crispy sage leaves. Mashing up cannellini beans with rosemary oil and shallots proved to be a winner, too. Keith and his wife tried giving Gracie pretty much anything they were eating: lentils milled with caramelized onions and wilted arugula or flaked white fish, stirring in ripe, fresh fruits (such as pears) or water or healthy oils (such as flax oil) to achieve a nice consistency. Keith even verified this approach with Dr. Bhatia, who liked the meal-sharing idea, as feeding a baby a range of foods encourages them to be more adventurous at the table.

This approach might not get everyone's approval. In fact, the American Academy of Pediatrics (AAP) warns parents against foods like spinach and against some home-prepared baby foods:

> *If you make your own baby food, be aware that home-prepared spinach, beets, green beans, squash, and carrots are not good choices during early infancy. They may contain large amounts of nitrates. Nitrates are chemicals that can cause an unusual type of anemia (low blood count) in young babies. Commercially prepared vegetables are safer because the manufacturers test for nitrates. Peas, corn, and sweet potatoes are better choices for home-prepared baby foods.*

The AAP guidelines are very cautious, particularly about vegetables. The first food the AAP mentions on its HealthyChild.org website is baby cereal. It does mention some vegetables (squash, peas, corn, carrots), but doesn't provide a specific list (and doesn't divide this list into age categories). When it provides a sample daily menu for an 8- to 12-month-old baby, it simply mentions "yellow or orange vegetables" and "green vegetables." Not specific enough to be helpful, in my opinion. And what about red vegetables, or purple ones?

In short, the advice from French and American pediatricians is contradictory, and American pediatricians don't agree with each other on the best approach to feeding babies. (The official AAP advice contradicts that of the FSP as well as Dr. Bhatia's views, even though he is a member of the AAP committee on nutrition.) Confusing, I know. But comparing the two approaches suggests you can probably be more ambitious about food diversification than the American guidelines suggest. My recommendation: do your own research and talk to your health-care provider about what makes sense for your family. Your health-care provider will also be able to give you the most up-to-date advice on allergies and on foods that you should delay introducing, such as eggs, shell-fish, unpasteurized honey, nuts, and citrus.

Whatever first foods you *do* serve to your baby, remember that it's best to wait a day after introducing each one to see if there are any allergic reactions. On **GettingToYum.com** you'll find sample food diversification menus for a 6-, 7-, and 8-month-old baby. By the time they're 9 months old, babies should be able to start eating the purée recipes that begin on page 181. If you add those in progressively, your child will be eating a broad range of vegetables by the time they are 2 years old.

It's worth noting that some researchers and pediatricians are increasingly questioning the North American approach to child feeding, particularly the emphasis on a limited variety of foods in the first year and the choice of processed white rice cereal as the first food for babies. Dr. David Ludwig, Director of the Optimal Weight for Life Program at the Boston Children's Hospital (one of the nation's leading obesity research centers), argues that conventional white rice baby cereal—which has had most of the vitamins and nutrients removed through processing—is the nutritional equivalent of table sugar. He argues that such foods raise blood sugar and insulin levels without providing nutrients (apart from the added iron). In other words, rice cereal—our North American mainstay—might just be among the worst foods for infants.

How is it possible that something so nutritionally bankrupt became a cornerstone of our infant diet? It may be because some rice cereals are iron-fortified, and iron is one of the few widespread nutritional deficiencies in the United States. However, there are other ways to provide iron, notably through naturally iron-rich foods (like spinach), provided they are served with a little vitamin C (found in tomatoes, for example) to help with absorption.

Are the infant and child-feeding guidelines currently recommended in North America, which often lead to children receiving the bulk of calories in the form of heavily processed rice cereal and other carbs, inadvertently training our children to prefer processed and junk food? Some doctors think so. Well-known pediatrician Dr. Alan Greene argues that the North American approach teaches children to prefer certain kinds of foods such as white bread, crackers, and pasta. By 18 months, few American toddlers are eating whole grains on a daily basis. Dr. Greene encourages parents to serve brown rice cereals instead (or homemade rice mash or vegetable purée) and has even launched a "White-Out Campaign" calling for an end to the recommendation of serving processed cereals—specifically white rice cereal—to babies (drgreene.com/whiteout). It may make sense to think twice about rice cereal.

When should I start taste training my baby?

AS SOON AS YOUR BABY STARTS EATING SOLID FOODS! IT'S RELATIVELY EASY at this stage, since most babies are naturally curious about new foods (just as they are with new toys). In fact, most babies will put everything into their mouths, food and non-food items alike (my older daughter even sampled rocks, gravel, and dirt!) Take advantage of their natural curiosity to get them sampling lots of different tastes—and not just bland tastes.

Recommendations for when to start solid foods vary between countries and depend in part when the recommendations were written. At the moment, 6 months seems to be the preferred age (introducing solid foods before the age of 4 months may raise the risk of allergies). Pediatric recommendations in some countries also suggest avoiding some foods (such as unpasteurized honey) until 12 months or older. Check the guidelines that are relevant to you, then consult with your pediatrician and specifically discuss any foods that may pose allergy risks for your child. Whenever you start, your goal should be to take advantage of your baby's natural curiosity about foods and to introduce lots of variety before they are 2 years old, when the picky eating phase begins for many children.

You should know, however, that there is no magical age at which babies are ready. Some babies will be interested earlier, some not. My first daughter was tremendously interested in food at the age of 4 months. My second daughter wasn't interested until later, and since she didn't have many teeth until quite late, she was slow to start chewing solid foods.

Each baby develops differently—your baby will be your best guide. They will let you know when they are ready! Some babies may mimic you eating, bringing their hand up to their faces. Others may grunt or gesture, and even try reaching for the food. When they do start eating, some babies may have trouble keeping the food in their mouths. At this age, their natural extrusion reflex may cause them to push food out of their mouth with their tongue. This natural protective mechanism will disappear after a few weeks or months at most.

Stick to simple, single-ingredient dishes for the first month or two, after which you can try introducing fun combinations. Babies can start eating herbs and spices at 9 months, which is why the purée recipes in the second part of this book contain ingredients like cinnamon, oregano, cumin, and basil. *Yum!*

Do I need any special equipment?

IN TERMS OF GEAR, I PERSONALLY BELIEVE LESS IS MORE. AT A MINIMUM, you'll probably find it helpful to have a high chair, an unbreakable baby spoon and bowl, bibs, and at least one device for puréeing food, whether it be a food mill, food processor, blender, or immersion blender. A BebeCook machine steams and purées all at once, and can even defrost. You can achieve the same results (and smoother purées) with a simple steamer insert for one of your pots and an immersion blender.

When and how do I feed my baby?

THERE IS NO MAGIC FORMULA OR ONE-SIZE-FITS-ALL RULE TO TEACHING your child to be a good eater, but the following are some tips that will work for most families.

Do create a schedule. It can be fluid and flexible, but create some notion of a schedule that includes three meals a day served roughly at the same times as your meals. Add scheduled snacks as appropriate. The FSP recommends one snack per day (in the mid-afternoon), whereas the AAP recommends three (mid-morning, mid-afternoon, and bedtime). A simple daily schedule might look like this: breakfast between 8 and 9 a.m., lunch between 12 and 1 p.m., snack at 3:30 p.m., and dinner between 5:30 and 6:30 p.m. Naptimes, illnesses, playdates, and other commitments will of course mean that you'll vary these times a bit. Not to worry! Whatever schedule you adopt, the point is to clearly distinguish eating times from non-eating times.

Don't try to control your baby's eating. It's your job to schedule meals and to present a good variety of food in a relaxed, comfortable setting. It's your baby's job to decide whether and how much they eat. Don't insist that they eat more if they're full, don't insist that they eat things they're refusing, and, above all, never force your baby to eat.

Do watch out for choking hazards, and for hot spots when rewarming food. Puréed foods are best for younger babies, and chewable foods, which are generally introduced between 10 and 12 months, should be offered cautiously at first. When transitioning babies to chewable foods, make sure the dishes are cooked until they can be easily squashed with a fork. Make bite sizes teeny-tiny (about the size of a raisin). An easy rule of thumb: any food placed in the child's mouth should be able to be swallowed as is, without chewing.

Do make variety a habit by rotating through foods regularly. If babies get used to novelty early on, they're less likely to develop a restricted favorite foods list as toddlers (only pancakes for breakfast, only pasta for lunch, and so on). Introduce as much variety as you can, in colors as well as flavors. Establish the expectation that novelty is normal.

Don't worry if your baby makes a mess. Of course babies will sometimes make a mess. How much mess you are willing to tolerate is up to you, but it's not a concern. If you do want your baby to eat tidily, it's certainly possible. Watching French babies taught me that babies can actually learn to eat relatively tidily, right from the start. For starters, they simply aren't allowed to play with their food. For example, throwing food means that the plate is removed (once and for all!) from the table, and even young babies quickly learn that if they're hungry they'd better not throw their carrot purée at the floor.

Do make homemade baby food. This can be fast and easy if you're organized. Freezing purées in large batches saves time, and you can also mix homemade with store-bought purées to introduce more taste variety. Committing to make homemade purées means that you'll have lots of fruits and veggies around—and eat more of them yourself, too. If you're worried about time not spent with your baby, put them in their high chair in the middle of the kitchen and give them some pots and pans and spoons to bang and play with. They'll have fun watching you "cooking," too!

Do eat everything your baby eats. Research shows that children are much more likely to try a new food if their parent tries it first—with obvious enjoyment. If it isn't tasty for you, then it might not be for your baby, either. Try new combinations; sometimes your baby may be ready for more interesting tastes, which will sustain their interest in foods.

Don't add extra salt to your baby's food. If you're serving your baby a portion of an adult dish, make sure to remove their portion before you add salt. Remember that babies have on average many more taste buds than adults. They'll enjoy the natural flavors without the salt.

Do steam veggies whenever possible. For meats and fish, any cooking method that retains moisture (such as poaching fish) is a good bet, as this will make it easier for babies to chew and swallow.

Do vary your cooking methods in order to give some taste variety. Steaming is best in terms of nutrient conservation, but you can also sauté in a little butter, olive oil, or canola oil (sautéed zucchini is delicious, for example, as are red peppers). Roasting is easy but time-consuming, and will intensify flavors (especially of yams, squash, and sweet potatoes). Roasting also allows you to prepare combinations of adult and baby veggies at the same time—just cut the veggies in large chunks, add water, and roast in the oven at 375°F until tender. Season and serve your portion, and purée your baby's portion. *Voilà!*

Don't get stuck in a rut. When making food combinations for your purées, don't be afraid to vary the quantities of the base ingredients. If the purée tastes slightly different each time, so much the better. Your baby will get used to more novelty.

Do offer finger foods as your child develops the "pincer grip" between forefinger and thumb some time between 10 and 12 months old. Be sure to slice any smooth foods (such as grapes or cherry tomatoes) into small pieces to avoid choking hazards. Small pieces of chopped-up veggies (such as green peas) or fruit (such as blueberries) make for great finger foods.

Don't be averse to a little fat in your child's food. Children need to eat a moderate amount of healthy fats for optimum growth and development. Fat helps with the absorption of fat-soluble nutrients. Plus, fat adds flavor. A dab of butter on spinach purée will make it that much more palatable. You can also use high-quality oils (such as olive oil) in moderation.

Do have your child sit at the table while eating. It's a good habit, if only for safety reasons: kids are less likely to choke when sitting calmly and focusing on chewing.

Do eat yourself at baby's mealtime. Babies are natural mimics, and it's an educational experience for them to sit with you at the table. As they see their older siblings and parents or caregivers trying new foods, they'll be more likely to try new things.

Do keep a diary of what your child is eating and their reactions. It will help you think about what to introduce next and remind you about including variety, plus you'll be able to see emerging patterns of likes and dislikes.

Don't allow emphatic expressions of food dislikes at your family table. Children are highly suggestible; if another child or adult declares that he or she doesn't like something, chances are your baby will follow suit. Teach your other family members to either say nothing or to politely say "no, thank you."

Don't assume your baby won't like something. Let them decide. If it's safe to eat, let them try it. And don't assume their food preferences will be like yours. That being said, your child will refuse to try foods, so prepare yourself for the inevitable.

What do I do when my baby refuses to try a new food?

FOOD REFUSALS CAN BE ONE OF THE MOST FRUSTRATING THINGS ABOUT parenting. They raise our anxiety levels and often feel like rejection. The most important thing (and I know this is hard to do): don't pressure your baby in any way. Simply remove the food without comment and do not offer a replacement or substitute. You don't want to fall into the trap of short-order cooking, and you don't want to reinforce the refusal behavior. Try offering the food again in a few days or a few weeks.

Feeding your baby is like a conversation. If you're sensitive to their cues, your baby will gain confidence. You'll avoid creating emotional associations with food, and your baby will learn the skill of eating at their own pace.

Remember that babies are acute tasters. They have more taste buds on average than adults. Babies can distinguish different kinds of sugars from one another—even at low concentrations. They can even distinguish their mother's breast milk from other's breast milk just a few days after being born. They are highly capable of tasting and enjoying the full range of flavors in all foods—all the more reason not to give them solely bland food (but it may take them a few tries to get used to it).

Following the vegetable rotation rule will help you deal with food refusals as well. Rotating vegetables frequently keeps things interesting (and later on, with toddlers, lowers tension at the table, particularly if you make sure your child is being served foods they like in between the "scary" foods). Of course, if you offer greater variety, you will find more things that your child does like, and you'll be less likely to create a battle of wills over foods that they don't like. Remember, learning to like vegetables is a matter of "practice makes perfect."

Another point to remember is that while each baby has their own distinct eating style, there are common developmental patterns most babies share. Most babies between the ages of 2 and 3 will show more negative reactions to food, become more distractible when eating (sound familiar?), and develop more unpredictable appetite patterns for a period of time. The emergence of negative food reactions is thought to be a normal developmental pattern, as babies start figuring out what they like (and don't like) and as their diet becomes more varied and diverse. Distractibility increases as children reach the age of 2, when their growth slows down and their appetite diminishes. Around this time, you'll probably also notice that your baby's appetite will become increasingly predictable (with regular times when they are hungry), as their eating style becomes apparent and as they start to adapt to your family's eating schedule.

At the same time, you'll start to learn more about your baby's individual eating style, which is evident even in babies as young as 6 months. Babies (just like adults) tend to exhibit one of three eating styles:

1. **The Easy Eater.** This type of eater (about 3 in 10 babies) has a more predictable appetite and is less distractible at mealtimes—basically, they're really interested in food, eager to get it, and won't let much get in their way if they're hungry. They're not fussy, usually calm at mealtimes, and generally open to new food experiences. Often, these children also

have a low emotional reactivity; they're the easygoing kids. My nephew Damien is this type of eater; he'll focus with single-minded intensity on getting the most food in as little time as possible. With Damien (as is sometimes the case with kids in this category), overeating is occasionally a concern.

2. **The Strong-Minded Eater.** This type of eater has a fairly predictable appetite, is somewhat (but not too) distractible at mealtimes, and has clear food preferences: likes and dislikes that emerge early and may intensify over time. This type of eater (approximately 5 or 6 out of 10 babies) is sometimes a handful, and sometimes reacts to new foods, but generally gets used to them over time. My younger daughter, Claire, is this type of eater—mostly happy to eat, but not afraid to express her likes and dislikes.

3. **The Reactive Eater.** These children (approximately 1 or 2 out of 10 babies) react very strongly to foods and tend to have a narrow set of preferred foods. They're often more distractible at mealtimes and have a less predictable appetite pattern; they may also be more anxious about eating and more emotionally reactive to food (and to things in general). These children are the most likely to be strongly neophobic (afraid of new foods) when they are toddlers, and it will take more time and persistence to help them learn to eat a varied diet. If this describes your child, I can empathize: my older daughter, Sophie, was a reactive eater. The days of her "crazy food dance" (in which she would roll her eyes, stamp her feet, and even jump up and down if presented with a food she didn't like) are long gone, but none of us had an easy time. With Sophie, as is sometimes the case with fussy eaters, getting her to eat enough food was sometimes a worry. (How long can a toddler survive on smoothies and buttered toast?)

Your baby has their own "eating personality" with traits as durable and long-lasting as other aspects of their personality. Your job is to figure out your child's eating style and encourage them to expand their palate while being respectful of their individual differences. Some babies will go more slowly than others, but don't give up hope. You *can* teach your child to eat—with the right combination of love and limits, persistence and perspective, encouragement and common sense.

Toddlers: Preventing and Solving Common Eating Challenges

FEEDING TODDLERS AND PRESCHOOLERS IS OFTEN FRUSTRATING. ANXious to make sure their children are getting enough nutritious food, parents are often confronted with children with strong taste preferences who want to eat the same foods nearly every day (often the more unhealthy foods in the family repertoire).

Parents know what to feed their toddlers (usually, more fruits and vegetables), but they don't know *how* to get them to eat those healthy things. Many toddlers prefer bland foods (things made with white refined flour, such as crackers and bread) to anything else. I know this from personal experience: when she was 2, my oldest daughter would have eaten nothing but pasta and buttered toast if we'd let her. Many of my test families reported something similar. This, of course, is developmentally normal: whereas babies are exploring yet closely attached, toddlers are becoming little individuals—at times resisting parents while exploring their individuality and newfound sense of power.

As a result, few toddlers and preschoolers eat the recommended five servings of fruits and vegetables a day. Their eating patterns are often unpredictable; sometimes they seem very hungry; other times they seem completely uninterested in food. The USDA recommendation that *half* your plate should be fruits and vegetables (at every meal!) can seem almost laughable when confronted with the fickle, finicky tastes of younger children.

Despite all of this, my main message is still *don't worry*. If your child's height and weight are within the normal range according to your health-care provider, and if your child looks healthy and is usually happy and full of energy, then their picky eating behaviors are likely just a normal phase of development. There are, however, some warning signs to look out for. If your child seems to have trouble chewing, regularly refuses most foods, does not have regular bowel movements that are soft and easy to pass at least once every day or two, urinates less than four times per day, is not sleeping 10 to 12 hours per night, and is not eating at least one item from each of the main food groups—fruits, vegetables, grains, proteins (such as meat, fish, beans, nuts, and seeds), dairy (or substitutes), and healthy fats and oils—a day, then you should consult your health-care practitioner.

In most cases, your child's picky eating habits are likely to be completely normal. Your worries about your child's eating habits are also normal. Many parents are concerned that their child eats too many unhealthy foods (such as refined white flour, sugar, processed foods), doesn't eat enough healthy foods (vegetables, proteins, and whole grains typically feature high on this list), or simply doesn't eat enough, period. You're not alone! Picky eating is a developmental phase, and most children will need your guidance in order to overcome it. Remember: you can teach a child to eat just like you teach them to read—but they do need regular practice and your guidance.

Creating healthy boundaries—using the simple routines and rules introduced in the Seven Secrets—is an important part of this guidance. *How* and *when* kids eat (for example, with a structured routine of three meals and one or two snacks per day) helps with *what* kids eat. Remember your routine, and stick to it.

Another important strategy is to adapt your meals slightly (just ever so slightly) to your toddler's developing eating abilities. Here are some key tips:

- Make sure your child is comfy: feet propped up and with good back support. Believe it or not, toddlers' chewing effectiveness depends on how well their core is supported—by their feet! Prop up their feet with firm support.
- Make food physically easy to eat (meat is soft and moist; salad is cut up as finger food).
- Serve small servings: allow your child to ask for more, but don't serve them too much at the start.
- Serve veggies or fruit first, preferably at both lunch and dinner.

A little cautionary note: the rules and routines aren't meant to make mealtimes overly rigid. Toddlers learn to eat best when their parents are relaxed. If you start early enough and are persistent enough, by the time your child is school-age (around 6 years old), they'll be eating more or less like an adult. You'll have introduced a range of textures and tastes into your child's diet and helped them learn a structured eating routine. Food will increasingly be a source of fun for the whole family (and not a cause for food fights).

Along the way, though, you're likely to encounter three challenges. Many toddlers have difficulty:

1. Accepting different textures
2. Mixing foods (and eating "mixed" dishes)
3. Interpreting and coordinating signals from different senses (sight, hearing, touch, smell, and taste) when encountering new foods

Below are some simple tips and tricks to help you overcome these challenges.

The toddler texture challenge

TODDLERHOOD IS THE STAGE WHEN CHILDREN BEGIN ENCOUNTERING—AND mastering—different textures. Chewing seems so natural to adults that it is easy to forget this is a big step up from babyhood. Think of how difficult it must be to learn to like crunching hard foods. I still have a very clear memory of how proud my older daughter was when she first munched through a raw carrot—no mean feat, given those little teeth and that little jaw!

Discomfort with textures is a common problem for toddlers, and it's often an important reason they enjoy (or reject) foods. Part of the reason is mechanical: toddlers' teeth and jaws (as well as the surrounding muscles) are still developing, and so it may be difficult for them to be in full control of certain foods in their mouths. Toddlers will tend to reject textures that are difficult to manipulate in their mouths (and rightly so, from their perspective). Vegetables, with their slippery, slimy textures (like mushrooms) or hard, crunchy textures (which some kids find difficult), or (even worse) combined soft and slippery textures (raw tomatoes), are literally hard for kids to get their teeth into.

Toddlers' suspicion of textures is thus at least partially a natural protective mechanism against the risk of choking. Although choking is indeed a risk (see the next page), you'll want to help your child figure out which textures they *can* eat without risk. The texture play aspect of the games and experiments listed here will help you do just that.

The simplest approach of all is to adapt the textures of the foods you are serving to suit your toddler's evolving skills. Here are some examples:

- If your child is starting to learn to eat lettuce, try ripping it into very small pieces or serving only the hard spine of the lettuce leaves, which is crunchier and more like the apples, carrots, and celery they might already be enjoying.
- Make sure that any meat you serve is cut into very small morsels and is seriously tender and moist. Often, an aversion to meat is a rejection of texture (and the demands of chewing), not a rejection of the taste. See page 30 for tips.
- Turn texture into a game in its own right. In our house, we invented the Carrot Crunch variation of Game 13: Terrific Textures (page 100) to encourage our younger daughter to eat crunchy carrots. Preschoolers are playful and love to imitate parents. Take advantage of those tendencies.

Gagging versus choking

GAGGING IS A NORMAL SWALLOWING REFLEX THAT PREVENTS CHOKING: when food slips to the back of the mouth, gagging pushes it forward again. Knowing that, try to remember that if you don't react to your child gagging, they won't either. They'll continue eating. Just calmly explain that gagging is no reason to worry, and teach them how to avoid it by taking small mouthfuls and chewing properly.

Choking is, of course, dangerous. If a child is able to breathe, or cough, they will probably expel the food item themselves. But if a child is making no sound or only a squeaky, whistling sound, they may be choking. Choking tends to happen when you breathe in at the same time as you swallow. The risk is higher with slippery foods (such as hot dogs, sausages, grapes, baby carrots—foods that are just the right size to clog up the windpipe) and with foods that are tough to chew (such as steak, hard nuts, or candies) or sticky (such as large globs of peanut butter). Make sure to protect your child by avoiding the above-mentioned foods before the age of 3 and chopping up foods after that age (for instance, cut grapes into quarters). Encourage your child to be calm at the table and to eat only when seated. Most important, have your health-care provider teach you basic first aid for choking.

Mixing textures

MANY CHILDREN DON'T LIKE MIXING DIFFERENT TEXTURED FOODS TOGETHER. This is completely normal and a passing phase. Part of the reason is simply that toddlers are still learning to chew and manipulate foods in their mouths, and mixing textures makes this more complicated. Another reason is that kids are still learning (and shuffling) cognitive categories at this age. For example, if you serve carrots in a slightly different way (say, sprinkled with parsley rather than the plain style they're used to), kids may see this as an entirely new dish. This is why they're sometimes happy to eat certain foods on their own, but not mixed together. A classic example: 3-year-old Tobias, the son of one of my test families, liked red peppers and scrambled eggs, but serve him an omelet with red peppers in it and he'd refuse to eat it.

The solution? Put your child in charge, as my test families did, with great results:

> *Tobias doesn't like things combined . . . unless he gets to mix them himself. I think it gives him a sense of control, because I've noticed that if he gets to do the mixing, there's no problem. So if I'm introducing him to a new food, I now get him to help me make the dish. We made an omelet together last week, which was an experiment because he doesn't really like omelets (although he's actually really good at breaking eggs and can crack them single-handed without getting any shells in the bowl!). We added peppers and spinach and lots of cheese, and we watched it all bubble up together. It was so nice, for both of us. This was after a long day of work, so cooking together served as quality time as well as my time to make dinner. And he ate it and said it was delicious. Sometimes for lunch or on lazy evenings I give him a piece of pita bread and let him fill it with cucumbers and cheese or leftover chicken or steak—so long as he's doing the adding, he's fine with it.*
>
> —MARTHA

Three-year old Tobias's experience is typical of many kids his age. Different textures combined in a single dish are often challenging for young children. But you can help your child get over this fear. Game 16: The Mixing Game (page 118) develops this idea into a set of sequenced games that will help your child get used to the idea of mixing textures.

Taste and texture testing

THE TODDLER STAGE IS WHEN THE TASTE-TESTING APPROACH BECOMES YOUR best friend. For cautious toddlers, visual exposure *prior* to taste testing can have really positive effects. This might include showing a vegetable, fruit, or dish to your child, allowing them to handle the ingredients, or reading books about food out loud (you'll find a list of some great children's books with positive messages about food on **GettingToYum.com**).

Remember: you can use taste testing to explore textures as well as tastes. If you think you're too busy to organize taste testing, try incorporating it into your daily cooking routine. Before you mash the potatoes, set one aside; serve a slice of boiled potato along with the mashed potatoes and ask your child to compare the two. Or use the rotation rule to help you explore textures: serve carrots raw one day, parboiled the next, in a soup the day after. Taste testing isn't complicated or time-consuming, but it does require you to be attentive and a little inventive. Above all, try to avoid "sneaky chef" strategies. They're nutritionally okay, but developmentally questionable. Keep offering your child opportunities to learn to eat the "scary foods"—the more frequently (and calmly) you do so, the more quickly they'll come around.

The games your toddler might play with you

TODDLERS LOVE TO TEST BOUNDARIES AND PUSH BUTTONS, AND ARE JUST beginning to explore what power struggles are all about. They're really like little psychologists, trying to figure out what they can get away with and whether they can get a reaction (happiness, anger, fear, annoyance) out of others. This experimentation is normal, but can also be scary for toddlers. They do want firm boundaries and will respond well when these are in place, as Hélène, mother of 18-month-old Pablo, found out:

> *A recent challenge was when Pablo discovered one of his many superpowers: taking off his bib in the middle of the meal. I had originally established a rule that we must wear a bib and sit in the high chair to eat. When he discovered I was annoyed when he was taking off his bib, he started doing it repeatedly, very early in the meal, and would push me into a power struggle. I fell into that trap a couple of times and then realized my error. A power struggle was making the situation worse, and it was ruining my meal, as I would get upset. And he wouldn't eat any more anyway. So I thought, okay, just go with a simple, calm consequence.*
>
> *The next time he took off his bib mid-meal, I said nonchalantly, "Okay, you are done with eating? Fine by me." (I was thinking to myself, if he's*

hungry, he'll eat better at the next meal.) And I let him leave the table, while we continued to eat our meal. The first couple of times I did this, he was pretty surprised and hung out near us, trying to get our attention. After about four times, he stopped taking off his bib during the meal. Now, at the end of the meal, he points to it, saying "Maman" with his sweet voice and signing "please," to ask if he can take off his bib. I ask him if he's finished eating, and if he's not, we go on with the meal. If he is, so be it. I was relieved this worked!

—HÉLÈNE

Remember: children may decide to test your rules and routines, particularly if you are implementing them when they're a bit older. A child may decide to misbehave at the table; if so, you might have to ask them to leave and be firm about them not coming back to finish the meal or be with the family, explaining that they can try again at the next meal. A toddler may repeatedly try to remove their bib; if so, firmly signal that their meal is over. If you're firm, they'll quickly learn.

A common way young children will test boundaries is with the "I won't eat" tactic. My younger daughter tried this on us when she wasn't quite 3 years old. "I *won't* eat," she announced one dinnertime. "Fine," we said. "It's bedtime, so you can go upstairs and go to bed." "*Fine!*" she huffed and dramatically stormed (well, as much as a 3-year-old can storm) up to her bedroom. We said nothing and happily continued on with our meal. Within 5 minutes, she had come back to the table, settled in, and started eating. We didn't make a big deal of it, and it never happened again.

A variation on the previous tactic is the "I'm not hungry" strategy. It may very well be that your child is not hungry (did they have a big piece of cake at a birthday party in the late afternoon?), but they also may just be trying to push your buttons. Here's one approach that Ellyn Satter, a doyenne of American nutrition writers, recommends: simply say "You don't have to eat, but come and keep us company for a few minutes." If they choose to leave: "Fine, but that is all until your next mealtime." If they come back to the table to eat, let them do so without much comment. If they fuss, don't get angry (you're paying them attention, and thus rewarding them). If you're firm, your child will probably only try this gambit on you once.

Other strategies have been covered in earlier chapters:

- **"I don't like that!"** The "veggies first" and "you just have to taste it" rules help you deal with the inevitable "I don't like that" responses.
- **"I want pasta!"** Remember, you've committed to avoiding short-order cooking, so no pasta (or whatever else they may be demanding) on short notice if they don't like what they see on the table. It's exhausting for you and doesn't offer opportunities for your child to learn. At our house we like the motto "You get what you get, and you don't get upset." Make sure there is something they like on the table (like bread) that they can eat if they really don't want to eat anything else.

"Look at me, Mommy!" A more subtle game sometimes revolves around praise: children exaggerate good (or alternate good and bad) behavior in order to get praise from adults. A simple way to avoid this is to not give excessive praise. You can comment if they eat well, but don't go over the top, and don't praise for behavior that's ordinary (or should be ordinary). The important thing is that *they* are proud of themselves; it's not *your* issue. The dinner-table conversation should not revolve around your child's eating habits; as explored in Secret 4: Routines and Rituals Make Healthy Eating Automatic (and Fun) (page 75), there are other "table talk" strategies that you can use.

Keep it positive! Balancing love and limits

TODDLERS HAVE A LOT TO LEARN ABOUT EATING, AND THERE'S A LOT TO remember as a parent. Ultimately, it's all about striking a healthy balance between love and limits. At times, you'll want to be firm; at other times, try a lighter touch. In general, you're probably being too controlling if you make your child clean their plate, eat all of their food before dessert, stay at the table (after everyone else has left) to finish their food, or only let them eat three meals a day (kids do need at least one snack). On the other hand, you're probably not setting strong enough limits if you short-order cook or produce special food for your child at many meals, let your child have snacks (or juice or milk) whenever they want, allow your child to behave badly at the table, or bribe your child with food to do basic tasks (like get in the car or put his clothes on in the morning). Creating good routines now will serve you well for a lifetime.

REMEMBER THOSE ROUTINES!

The toddler years are the best time to establish healthy eating practices. Suggestions include:

- Schedule meals and snacks (and stick to it).
- Eat at the table and nowhere else (no chasing a distractible toddler around the house with a spoon and a bowl—if for no other reason than it's a choking hazard).
- Avoid pressure at the table: no catering, forcing, bribing, cajoling, enticing.
- Kids eat what adults eat: no short-order cooking and no substitutes.
- Follow the variety rule: introduce one new food per day (or per week or whatever time period suits your family). Trust me: novelty will work for you rather than against you. This is your way of giving your toddler the opportunity to learn to eat new foods.
- Follow the rotation rule: serve new foods or old favorites in new ways, every single day.
- Parents provide, kids decide: be appropriately encouraging about tasting new foods, but let your toddler decide what they do and don't eat.
- Create rituals: table talk rituals, politeness rules—if you instil them now, things will be much, much easier when they're older. Really!

Establishing routines like these sets the stage for learning new tastes and textures: your toddler will come to meals hungry, in a positive mindset, and ready to behave reasonably well when at the table.

School-Age Children: Smart Strategies for Raising Food-Savvy Kids

R AISING HEALTHY EATERS TAKES A DIFFERENT TURN WHEN YOUR children are school-age. They're now spending more time in environments beyond parental control, exposed to the pressures of school food offerings and marketing. The landscape they're negotiating is much more complex—luckily, they're old enough to start learning the skills they need.

As explored in Secret 2: Marketing Healthy Food to Your Kids Really Works, children need the ability to decipher the marketing messages they encounter everywhere around them—particularly on TV and online, but also at school. The American Academy of Pediatrics (AAP) recommends no screen time for kids under the age of 2, and only 1 to 2 hours per day for older kids (the average is 4 hours per day).

An equally powerful strategy is counter-marketing, which provides your kids with the skills to decipher and resist marketing messages. Kids have to be aware that ads surround them and be able to identify them. They need to understand what the ads are trying to do, and they need to be motivated to resist the advertising.

As discussed in Secret 2, counter-marketing isn't purely defensive. You can market healthy food to your kids, too. Some of the games and experiments listed in this chapter are designed to help you do "positive marketing" by making healthy food fun and interesting for kids. Sound crazy? Think back to Game 5: The Silly Name Game on page 52. Kids' consumption of vegetables went up by as much as 100 percent when parents and teachers gave playful names to dishes. We do this all the time at our house. Would you rather eat pearl barley or Fairy Baguette? An avocado smoothie or a Monster Smoothie?

For older kids, this is no less important, but your "marketing" techniques—as shown here—will become more subtle. Encourage your tween and adolescent children to develop food preferences and tastes as part of their exploration of individual identity. One of my test family parents, for example, was thrilled that their teenage son discovered a love of green beans; he even ended up cooking them regularly for his family. This is another important point: many teenagers will also develop an interest in cooking food for themselves as part of their journey toward independence.

In addition to marketing, the other key strategy at this age is *modeling* good eating behaviors. Continue with the healthy routines you've already set up (or create them now): three meals and one snack per day. Your older children may seem to need the family meal less (or may even complain about having to join you every day), but they need it just as much as they did when they were younger. They may even enjoy helping you prepare and cook food. In fact, one of the best ways to help a child learn to like new foods is to have them prepare it. They might even be interested in keeping a food-discovery diary, or researching fruits and vegetables.

As you model these healthy habits, keep in mind an important goal: helping your child to develop their own informed judgment about food and eating habits. Don't forget that your child is still developing skills. Some children are even continuing to develop fine motor skills by holding cutlery, and cutting and moving food from their plates into their mouths. Children also learn to multitask: listening to and participating in a conversation while eating is a valuable skill they'll have for life.

Neither modeling nor marketing imply that you're making all of the decisions for your child. If you're too controlling, your child will likely either completely rebel or depend too much on you to tell them what to do; either way, they won't develop their own judgment. You need to have informed discussions about marketing and the ways in which the manufacturers of processed foods try to manipulate our senses to get us to consume more. Some of the experiments in this chapter help you do just that. But the best way to explore these issues is to discuss them regularly. A regular family meal (whether breakfast or dinner, once a day or once a week) provides the best setting to do that. Building on the lessons, games, and experiments in Secret 5: Kids Don't Need Kids' Food (or going back and doing these, if you're reading this book by the time your children are school-age) will help your children learn sensory awareness and discuss their reactions to food, which helps them understand (and expand) their food preferences.

Remember, school-age children (particularly teenagers) are exploring and experimenting, which is natural and normal for their age. Luckily, their caloric needs are such that they can eat all the nutritious foods they need and still have a little room for some nutritionally marginal foods. If your child happily eats the healthy foods you provide at home while getting occasional treats at friends' houses or through using their allowance to buy snacks, then don't get too worried. Keep the big picture in mind: if they enjoy and eat nutritious foods, and are relatively happy with their body image, and if they're responding well to your parenting combination of love and limits, then they're on the right track. If not, you might need to make some adjustments to your routines, along with trying the experiments and games in this chapter.

Most important, remember that letting children make their own choices, in an age-appropriate way, is the best way to foster healthy eating habits. Parents who overtly control what their children eat are also more likely to have kids that are externally cued eaters (who eat in response to food cues such as the sight and smell of food, whether or not they're hungry) or emotional eaters (who eat in response to emotional rather than physical needs). These types of eaters are more likely to become obese. More subtly (particularly in the case of girls), children may develop a seesaw love/hate, restrictive/binging eating style.

This doesn't mean that parents shouldn't exert influence on what their children eat. Rather, they need to look for different methods: encouraging, teaching, and modeling (positive), rather than controlling (negative). Research suggests that strategies of covert control, in which parents control the child's food intake in a way that can't directly be detected by a child is a better strategy. At its simplest, this means creating a positive food environment for your child, in which healthy foods are essentially the only choice on a day-to-day basis. This might mean choosing to avoid restaurants that sell unhealthy foods, establishing a "no processed food" rule for grocery shopping, or creating a "once in a while treat" list, but otherwise serving mostly unprocessed foods at home. If these are family routines, then children are less likely to question them. This "covert control" actually increases children's consumption of healthy snacks and is associated with reduced obesity risk.

Even covert control goes only so far. What about when your child is in high school, with McDonald's just around the corner at lunchtime? Hopefully you'll have embraced your child's growing autonomy while shaping their ability to make good food choices. You want to develop what psychologists term a sense of "coherence" about food: a feeling of confidence (which arises through predictable routines and good boundaries) and a mixture of optimism and self-control (which comes through children exercising growing autonomy). This is the fine balance you're trying to strike: parents share a degree of control with kids, which evolves as your child develops.

Older Kids: Top Tips for Turning Picky Eaters into Easy Eaters

1. **Create a "new food challenge."** Get your child to pick a food they don't like, but that they know one of their friends or family members does like. Ask the two of them (helped by you if necessary) to come up with a recipe for that food item, which they can help prepare and serve to the family. The challenge: to convince the child who originally identified the "yucky" food that they might actually eat it. If that's too complicated, ask each child to pick a food they would like to be able to eat. Serve it different ways, every couple of days over a couple of weeks, and tell them that it will take between 7 and 12 tasting sessions before they probably learn to like it. Just like learning to ride a bicycle, your child needs practice.

2. **Practice the "one family, one meal" rule.** Involve your child in creating menus, using ground rules (for example, one fresh veggie every meal), and then stick to it. For example, work out a menu schedule on the weekend. Then, at meals during the week, use the "You don't have to eat it, but you do have to taste it" rule if your child is really being difficult. Use logical consequences (this is not a punishment!): for example, "If you don't finish your [small] serving of vegetables, no dessert."

3. **Involve your child in planning a meal celebration.** Get your child to help pick recipes, shop, cook, and prepare food for a family event (or dinner with guests at your house) during which they receive praise from others (not just you) for doing so.

4. **Try positive peer pressure.** Does your child have any friends or cousins (or know slightly older kids—that often works wonders!) who eat better and who would come over for a meal at your house to lead by example? Ask your visitor to suggest one of their favorite recipes in advance; if they eat it with gusto, there's a greater chance your child will, too.

5. **Try the Crunch a Color game.** Check out crunchacolor.com.

6. **Create a tasting week.** Ask each family member to pick a new food they'd like to learn to eat. Allow them to choose their preferred recipes; interested kids can help buy, prepare, and/or serve the foods to the entire family. Kids will enjoy turning the tables by picking a food that they know one of their parents doesn't particularly like!

A Final Thought: Get Rid of Guilt

I F YOU'RE READING THIS BOOK, IT'S BECAUSE YOU CARE ABOUT HELPING your child eat better. Please, put aside any blame you might have. You and your child are simply doing your best, and I hope that this book contains ideas that will help you reach your goals.

Putting aside blame also means removing guilt from the family food equation—for both you and your child. Don't label foods as good and bad. Rather, teach your child that there are foods that we eat regularly and foods that we eat occasionally. Equally, don't fall into the trap of forcing your child to eat "bad-tasting" food because it's "good for you." Instead, your goal should be to teach them to love the interesting flavors of all sorts of food.

Think of how your approach to food might change if you adopted this view. How would you teach your child the difference between, say, broccoli and chocolate? You might say this: "Chocolate tastes good. And, of course, broccoli does, too. But chocolate is a 'we eat this once in a while' food, while broccoli is a 'we eat this regularly' food." This approach means that kids don't grow up feeling guilty about liking bad-for-you (but good-tasting) foods, and they run a lower risk of developing unhealthy emotional (craving-indulgence-guilt-deprivation-fueled) eating behaviors later in life. This is really important for all children, but especially for toddlers, who may confuse the "food is bad for you" message with "I'm bad" messages, creating a food-guilt association that's hard to shake.

The simple message is this: try to have a positive rather than punitive attitude to food. Fear (of obesity, of not getting enough nutrients) shouldn't be our primary motivation for eating well. Guilt and anxiety shouldn't be our primary emotional associations with food. Your child isn't learning that we eat healthy food because we *have* to, but rather because we *want* to. That's how they—and your entire family—will develop positive food habits that will last a lifetime.

Getting to Yum Games

H ere's a reminder of the games you can play with your kids to instil positive food habits.

Game	Page	What the game teaches	Age level
1. The Five Senses	33	Taste is influenced by the five senses: sight, touch, hearing, smell, and taste. Kids will better understand their reactions to foods (both ones they like, and ones they don't like).	4 and up
2. The Five Flavors	34	The five different flavors: sweet, salty, sour, bitter, and *umami* (savory).	4 and up
3. Tasty Taste Buds	35	The science behind our taste buds, which are just like muscles: they can be trained!	4 and up
4. The Supertaster Game	37	We all experience taste differently. It may take correspondingly more (or less) time to learn to like new foods.	6 and up

Game	Page	What the game teaches	Age level
5. The Silly Name Game	52	Labeling foods can incite kids' enthusiasm for new food.	3 and up
6. The Smell-Taste Experiment	53	Smell plays a large part in determining how things taste. Artificial flavors are used to fool our taste buds.	6 and up
7. The Mystery Smell Game	54	Smell evokes emotions and memories, and affects our feelings about and perceptions of food.	6 and up
8. The Store-Brand versus Name-Brand Blind Taste Test	55	Brands influence (and can even fool) our sense of taste.	9 and up
9. The Sour Fruit Game	68	Sour is an "interesting" rather than a "yucky" taste.	2 and up
10. The Surprise Sack Game	69	Surprise introduces an element of fun to new foods at snack-time.	3 and up
11. The Smiley Face Game	85	A simple happy face makes eating more enjoyable.	1 and up
12. The Rose, Thorn, and Bud Game	86	A great ritual for keeping kids entertained at the table.	5 and up
13. Terrific Textures	100	Textures are more complex when foods are combined. Kids will learn to appreciate "adult" textures.	3 and up
14. The Color Confusion Experiment	104	Color influences our sense of taste.	6 and up

15. The Yogurt Game	105	Our sense of taste can be fooled by artificial coloring.	6 and up
16. The Mixing Game	118	This game teaches your child to enjoy different textures, and to develop their mixing skills, so they'll eat foods with combined textures more easily.	2 and up
17. Make-Your-Own Kids' Salad	120	This child-led cooking strategy helps kids overcome a common food dislike: salad. Many of my test families' kids were converted to salad lovers using this game.	4 and up
18. The Slow Food Experiment	131	The pace at which we eat our food influences how much we enjoy it. In general, the slower we eat, the better.	6 and up
19. The Same Food Three Ways Experiment	132	Food can taste dramatically different depending on preparation style.	4 and up
20. The Taste of Place Game	134	The concept of *terroir*, a French word that roughly translates as "taste of place."	6 and up

Recipes for Raising an Adventurous Eater

The Flavor-Ladder Approach

THESE RECIPES ARE SIMPLE BUT TASTY, WITH CLASSIC FLAVOR combinations: carrot purée gets a touch of dill, squash is paired with sage, green beans are matched up with almonds, and so on.

These dishes are also **quick to make:** they take, on average, 10 minutes to prepare. They are designed to reinforce the idea of **one family, one meal:** every recipe is designed for adults to enjoy along with their kids. This means healthy eating for the whole family and less work for you—no more short-order cooking!

Most important, these recipes are designed to enable you to teach your child to like eating a range of fruits and vegetables. They follow a simple "flavor-laddering" approach, **organized by age,** that **gradually introduces more complex tastes and textures as your child grows older.** Four different recipes are provided for each specific fruit or vegetable, one for each of the following four age groups:

Ⓐ Babies learning to eat solids

Ⓑ Older babies comfortable chewing soft foods

Ⓒ Toddlers (2½ or 3 years and up)

Ⓓ School-age kids (and kids of all ages)

By the time your child is ready for school, they should be ready to eat like a grown-up. If you have older children, don't worry: you can start them on any rung of the ladder at any time. Even the baby recipes—many of which are simple soups—are designed to be eaten and enjoyed by kids and adults of all ages.

INTRODUCING NEW FOODS TO BABIES: THE ISSUE OF ALLERGIES

The issue of when and how to introduce potentially allergenic foods is a matter of ongoing debate, and pediatric advice varies between countries. Consult your pediatrician before introducing your baby to solid foods, particularly if you or someone in your family has a history of food allergies or asthma. After you've consulted with your pediatrician, create a plan for adding new foods to your baby's diet, allowing time to monitor for a reaction to each specific food. To play it safe, and as per United States FDA recommendations, the following recipes for babies do not use honey, raw eggs, processed meats, unpasteurized cheeses, or any of the most allergenic foods for babies under the age of 12 months: milk, eggs, peanuts, tree nuts (such as almonds, walnuts, and pecans), soybeans, wheat, fish, or shellfish (such as crab, lobster, and shrimp).

Top 10 Veggies

THESE RECIPES ARE A GREAT PLACE TO START YOUR TASTE TRAINING. The "transition dishes" are perfect for picky eaters, but also designed to be tasty for adults. When you're ready, you can graduate to the next step: exploring more adventurous tastes in the "eating like a grown-up" category.

Top 10 veggies	Soup/purée 9 months and up	Starting solids 12 months (or whenever chewing soft foods) and up	Transition dishes—for grown-ups, too! 2½ to 3 years and up	Eating like a grown-up! 5 years and up (or whenever your child is ready)
Broccoli	George's Broccoli Purée (page 181)	Mollie's Enchanted Broccoli Rainforest (page 182)	Party Pasta (page 183)	French Minestrone Soup (page 185)
Carrots	Tasty Orange Trio (page 188)	Mae West Mash (page 189)	Vicious Carrots (page 190)	Grated Carrot Salad (page 191)
Cauliflower	Yummy Yellow Purée (page 194)	Marvelous Mashed Cauliflower (Faux Mashed Potatoes) (page 195)	Cauliflower Gratin (page 196)	Jeweled Cauliflower Rice (page 197)

Green Beans	Green Machine Purée (page 200)	Nifty Niçoise Soup (page 201)	Green Beans Amandine (page 202)	Salad Niçoise (page 203)
Peas	Minty Green Purée (page 207)	Eat Yer Greens Soup with Fresh Mint Cream (page 208)	Easy No-Stir Pea Risotto (page 209)	Chicken and Pea Curry (page 211)
Peppers	Roasted Red Pepper and Tomato Soup (page 214)	Red Rocket Hummus (page 215)	Pinwheel Pepper Wraps (page 216)	Ratatouille (Southern French Stew) (page 217)
Spinach	Note: In some countries, spinach isn't recommended for the youngest babies, due to the potential for high nitrate levels.	Sophie's Spinach Surprise (page 221)	Speedy Salmon Spinach Lasagna (page 222)	Warm Spinach Citrus Salad (page 224)
Squash	Squish Squash (page 227)	Roast Squash with Maple Cinnamon Sauce (page 228)	Squash Sage Soup (page 229)	Mild Thai Squash Curry (page 230)
Tomatoes	Tomato Peach Basil Purée (aka Baby Gazpacho) (page 233)	Rockstar Ragout (page 234)	Peek-a-Boo Stuffed Tomatoes (*Tomates Farcies*) (page 235)	Tasty Tagine Casserole (page 236)
Zucchini	Melt-in-Your-Mouth Zucchini Purée (page 239)	Roasted Zucchini with Cumin (page 239)	Zucchini Flan (page 240)	Quick Zucchini-Ham Quiche (page 241)

BROCCOLI

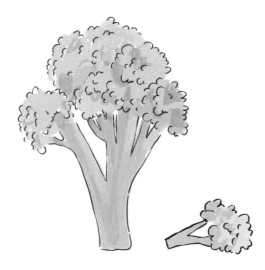

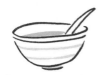
A GEORGE'S
BROCCOLI PURÉE

B MOLLIE'S ENCHANTED
BROCCOLI RAINFOREST

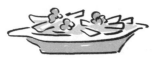
C PARTY PASTA

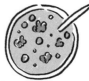
D FRENCH MINESTRONE SOUP

George's Broccoli Purée

11 minutes to prepare (5 minutes hands-on); makes 3 to 4 baby jars

GETTING BABIES USED TO THE TASTE AND COLOR OF BROCCOLI WHEN THEY'RE still young is a great idea. It's one of the mildest green vegetables you can serve. In this recipe, it pairs well with sweet potato and carrot. The thyme or tarragon (optional) will bring out the flavor of both the carrot and broccoli, and the sweet potato adds richness. Don't be afraid to add the butter (or olive oil): it evens out the taste and makes this dish rich and satisfying. Even cautious babies will love this one!

½ cup peeled and chopped sweet potato
½ cup peeled and chopped carrot
½ cup small broccoli florets (no stems)
Pinch chopped fresh thyme or tarragon leaves, optional
Dab unsalted butter (or 1 teaspoon olive oil), optional
Pinch sea salt, optional

1. In a small saucepan over medium-low heat, bring 2 cups of water to a boil. Add the sweet potato, then top with the carrot. Do not stir. Cover, increase heat to high, and cook for 3 minutes. Add the broccoli, reduce the heat to medium-high, and cook for 3 minutes more, or until the vegetables are tender. Strain the vegetables, reserving the cooking liquid to make the purée.
2. Transfer the vegetables to a food processor (or use an immersion blender), add the thyme, if using, and purée, adding enough cooking liquid to create a smooth consistency (start with ¼ cup, adding more as needed). To serve, top with a dab of butter (kids love watching it melt) and a small pinch of sea salt (if the butter in unsalted), if desired.

My fascination with taste training is how it's transforming my own eating. My son (22 months) asked for seconds after a good first portion. I loved it, too. I previously hated broccoli and can now objectively say that it's a great-tasting food! —JENNIFER

My kids thoroughly enjoyed the purée. It was easy to make. I kept it nice and chunky and added thyme. After I added butter and sea salt, they inhaled it! —MEG

Ⓑ Mollie's Enchanted Broccoli Rainforest

25 minutes to prepare (5 minutes hands-on); serves 2 adults and 2 children (as a side dish)

THIS RECIPE IS A LITTLE HOMAGE TO MOLLIE KATZEN, AUTHOR OF *The Enchanted Broccoli Rainforest*. It's one of my favorite kids' cookbooks because of the way it approaches vegetables—as something fun, interesting, and exciting. I used this recipe to get my resistant younger daughter to start eating broccoli. She referred to them as "trees" for a while and would nibble daintily on the "leaves" (refusing to eat the "trunks"). Luckily this was a passing phase, helped by the fact that my husband likes broccoli stalks. After seeing him enjoy them for a while, she began eating each and every morsel.

1 head broccoli, cut into small florets (about 4 cups)
2 tablespoons olive oil
¼ cup finely grated Parmesan cheese
¼ cup dried breadcrumbs
Pinch chopped fresh thyme or tarragon leaves, optional
Sea salt and ground black pepper, optional
1 tablespoon fresh lemon juice
2 tablespoons orange juice

1. Preheat the oven to 375°F.
2. In a bowl, combine broccoli and oil and toss to coat. Transfer to a baking dish and add enough water to cover the broccoli halfway. Roast in the oven for 20 minutes, or until the broccoli is tender. Drain the broccoli and set aside (see Note).
3. In a bowl, combine the Parmesan, breadcrumbs, and thyme, salt, and pepper, if using.
4. In a small bowl, combine the lemon and orange juices. Just before serving, pour the lemon-orange juice mixture over the broccoli and toss to coat. Add the breadcrumb mixture and toss to coat well.

Note: For younger babies (up until about 18 months), you'll probably want to set aside several broccoli florets before roasting and boil them until extremely tender, 5 to 7 minutes (roasting will also work, but it will take a lot longer than 20 minutes). For the youngest babies, you can also skip the juice and breadcrumb mixtures in Steps 3 and 4; however, once babies start eating it, they'll love it!

When my kids were younger, I often served this dish with mashed potatoes or Marvelous Mashed Cauliflower (page 195), making a little mountain of mash and inserting the broccoli like trees—artfully arranged, they do look like a little forest!

This was a breeze to make. My 14-month-old gobbled it up, and my husband and I loved it.

—MARTHA

 ## Party Pasta

20 minutes to prepare (5 minutes hands-on); serves 2 adults and 2 children

I OFTEN SERVE THIS DELICIOUS DISH AT INFORMAL DINNER PARTIES (HENCE the name). The anchovies add a salty flavor that really livens up the broccoli without a fishy flavor, and their oily tang is balanced by the fresh taste of lemon. Plus, anchovies (like other small cold-water fish) are incredibly nutritious. Combining this with a kids' favorite—pasta—makes this a winner for most children.

This dish was one of the top five favorites among all my test families. It was a surprise to most of them, because the combination of broccoli and anchovy can be a little intimidating. Trust me, it's delicious. Here's the score from the kids at the Alphabet Academy, who taste tested many of the recipes in this book: 22 out of 25 tried it, 17 finished it all, and 15 asked for seconds. Believe me, it's *that* good!

8 ounces dried penne or farfalle pasta (about 4 cups)

½ head broccoli, cut into bite-size pieces (about 2 cups)

Juice of ½ lemon (about 1 tablespoon)

3 tablespoons olive oil

3 to 5 anchovies (double if you really like anchovies; see Notes)

¼ cup grated Parmesan cheese (fresh is best, but I often used the pre-grated kind)

¼ cup dried breadcrumbs, optional

Pinch crushed red pepper, optional (for the more adventurous eaters in the family)

1. Bring a large pot of water to a boil over medium-high heat. Add the pasta and cook according to the package instructions, until al dente. Strain the pasta, reserving the cooking liquid for the sauce.

2. Meanwhile, bring a medium saucepan half-filled with water to a boil over medium-high heat. Add the broccoli and cook until just tender, 4 to 6 minutes. Drain the broccoli, transfer it to a bowl, and toss it with the lemon juice.

3. While the broccoli is cooking, in a large skillet over medium-high heat, heat the oil. Add the anchovies and ¼ cup of the pasta cooking liquid. Sauté for 3 minutes, or until the anchovies soften and start to dissolve. Reduce the heat to low and cook until the liquid has reduced to a sauce, about 3 minutes.

4. Add the cooked pasta to the skillet with the anchovy sauce and toss to coat. Add the prepared broccoli and toss to coat well. Serve topped with the Parmesan, and breadcrumbs and crushed red pepper, if using.

Notes: Anchovies are preserved in brine and then canned in oil (my preference) or salt (too salty for my taste). If you do use anchovies packed in salt, rinse them well first.

If you are really unsure about anchovies, try using anchovy paste in this dish. Substitute 1 scant tablespoon anchovy paste per anchovy in the recipe.

If making this dish in advance, do not toss the lemon juice with the broccoli (it will turn brown over time). Instead, keep the broccoli and lemon juice separate, then just before serving toss them together and add to the pasta.

Broccoli is no biggie in this house, and my 21-month-old already eats it, but then I saw anchovies and I freaked out a little bit! I've never cooked with anchovies (I pictured heads and bones and then realized that's sardines), so this was definitely stepping outside my own comfort zone. I'm over my fear of anchovies now. —TERESA

My kids (ages 3, 5, and 7) loved it. The lemon adds a nice zing and really brings out the flavors. —ROBERTA

I was nervous about the anchovies: I've really never eaten them, and they just sounded gross to me. That's why I chose to make this dish. I feel like I need to let go of my own food hang-ups if I'm going to teach my kids to eat everything. And to my pleasant surprise, my three kids all ate this dish happily and without complaint! —STACY

French Minestrone Soup

40 minutes to prepare (20 minutes hands-on); serves 6 adults or many hungry children

THIS SOUP FEATURES *PISTOU* SAUCE, WHICH IS TRADITIONAL IN SOUTHERN France, where it is often served with pasta or spread on bread, as well as used as a flavoring in soups and stews. There are many variations, but the basic principle is a sauce made from basil, garlic, and olive oil and often combined with Parmesan (much like pesto, but without the pine nuts). The rich flavor makes this veggie-packed soup worthy as a main dish.

Pistou can be used in so many dishes that I've included it as one of my Friendly Flavors: Basic Recipes (see page 301). My favorite traditional dish is the Provençal *soupe au pistou*, a summer soup that includes vegetables like green beans, tomatoes, and zucchini.

In this minestrone recipe, the *pistou* is made with broccoli as well as basil, but without the garlic, making for a mild, tasty sauce that's somewhat creamier than the traditional version. The soup includes lots of yummy, healthy vegetables and even some pasta.

This soup travels well in thermoses (I send it in the kids' lunch bags), and the *pistou* freezes well (use ice-cube trays to make smaller servings you can easily thaw).

2 tablespoons olive oil

1 medium onion, diced, or 1 large leek, white part only, diced

2 carrots, peeled and diced

2 zucchini, diced

½ pound green beans, trimmed and cut into bite-size pieces

1 teaspoon dried thyme

1 cup frozen peas

1 cup chopped broccoli florets

1 cup small dried pasta (such as mini-macaroni or orecchiette)

One 14-ounce can navy, Great Northern, or cannellini beans, rinsed and drained

3 bay leaves

10 cups *Brodo* (page 301) or ready-to-use low-sodium vegetable broth

1 teaspoon sea salt, optional

Pistou (page 304) for serving

¼ cup sun-dried tomato paste or puréed sun-dried tomatoes, for serving

1. In a Dutch oven or large soup pot, heat the oil over medium-low heat. Add the onion and cook, stirring occasionally, until translucent, 3 to 5 minutes. Add the carrots, zucchini, green beans, and thyme. Increase heat to medium-high and cook, stirring often, for 5 minutes, or until just tender (no longer, since the veggies will cook further in the soup). Add the peas, broccoli, pasta, beans, bay leaves, *brodo*, and salt, if using. Increase the heat to high and bring the soup to a boil, then reduce the heat to medium and simmer until the pasta is cooked, 6 to 8 minutes. Discard the bay leaves.

2. Ladle the soup into individual bowls. To each bowl, add about 1 teaspoon *pistou* and a small spoonful of sun-dried tomato paste and stir gently (see Note).

Note: The addition of *pistou* and sun-dried tomato paste is amazing in this dish. I often place bowls of *pistou* and sun-dried tomato paste on the table, as some people like to add more as they continue to eat. We also spread the *pistou* on bread, to accompany the soup—just as the French do.

Taste-Training Tip: *Pistou* can be used as a replacement for pesto with pasta. Try serving green pasta at Halloween!

My kids aren't big fans of soups in general, but this was a hit! After they each tried a little taste of the pistou, *I put it on the center of the table and let them add it to the soup themselves. They all added it generously, and it seemed to make eating soup more fun for them.* —ROBERTA

I wouldn't have guessed that broccoli could have been turned into a pesto-style sauce with such a rich fragrance. Loved the sunflower seeds. Plus, such a healthy meal! I felt like a rock star when my family inhaled the healthiest stew I've ever made. Thanks so much for pushing my boundaries with these vegetables. —LORI

CARROTS

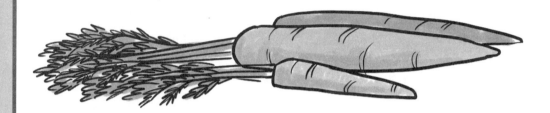

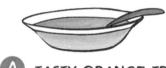

A TASTY ORANGE TRIO

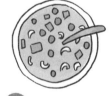

B MAE WEST MASH

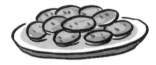

X-RAY VISION CARROTS!

C VICIOUS CARROTS

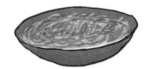

D GRATED CARROT SALAD

Tasty Orange Trio

13 minutes to prepare (5 minutes hands-on); makes 6 to 8 baby jars

CARROTS ARE A CLASSIC FIRST FOOD FOR BABIES, BUT THEY'RE OFTEN served plain. Not so in France! French parents introduce daily variations on familiar dishes to get their children used to new flavors, colors, and textures. Carrots, dill, and orange are a magical taste combination and often feature in adult soups. Parents can try this, too—you'll probably like it!

Once your baby is enjoying this purée, try substituting other herbs and spices for the dill, such as fresh parsley or cilantro or ground cumin. This is a great base from which to introduce your baby to lots of variety early on, so be inventive.

> 2 cups peeled and chopped carrots
> ½ cup orange juice
> ½ teaspoon dried dill

1. In a medium saucepan into which you have placed a steamer insert, bring 2 cups of water to a boil over high heat. Add the carrots to the steamer, cover, and steam until tender, about 8 minutes. If you don't have a steamer, simmer the carrots in water over medium-high heat for about 5 minutes. Strain the carrots, reserving the cooking liquid.
2. In a food processor, combine the cooked carrots, orange juice, and dill and purée, slowly adding enough cooking liquid to reach desired consistency. (Alternatively, you can use an immersion blender to purée the carrots in the pan.)

Note: This purée can easily be made the day before; the flavors intensify overnight. For adults or older kids, try adding more water to make a soup and season with a little grated ginger or cumin, plus salt, to taste.

Mae West Mash

20 minutes to prepare (5 minutes hands-on); serves 3 adults and 3 children

The only carrots that interest me are the number of carats in a diamond. —MAE WEST

THIS RECIPE USES THE CLASSIC FRENCH TRIO OF CARROTS, CELERY (OR celeriac), and onions (or leeks) known as *mirepoix*, which is used as the base for many French soups, stocks, and sauces. When served as a side dish (known as a *matignon*), the vegetables are gently sautéed in butter or olive oil over low heat, and herbs such as thyme are added. Set aside larger pieces of cooked vegetables as a perfect adult side dish for meat or lamb dishes, and gradually work your child up to an adult version of the mash they'll have come to love by leaving the purée more chunky as time goes on.

1 tablespoon olive oil or ½ tablespoon salted butter plus ½ tablespoon olive oil

1 cup diced leek, white part only, or diced onion

4 cups peeled and diced carrots

1 stalk celery, finely diced

½ cup water, *Brodo* (page 301), or ready-to-use low-sodium vegetable broth

2 bay leaves

¼ teaspoon dried thyme

1 cup cubed cooked ham, optional

1. In a large skillet over medium heat, heat the oil. Add the leek and sauté gently for about 3 minutes, until softened. Add the carrots and celery, increase the heat to medium-high, and cook for 3 minutes, stirring regularly. Add the water and bay leaves, increase the heat to high, and bring to a boil. Reduce the heat to medium, add the thyme, and simmer until the vegetables are tender and the liquid has evaporated, about 8 minutes. If using the ham, stir it in after 5 minutes. Remove the pan from the heat, discard the bay leaves, and serve—as is for older children and adults, or mashed for baby.

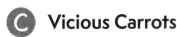

Vicious Carrots

25 minutes to prepare (5 minutes hands-on); serves 2 adults and 3 children

WHILE THE PROPER NAME FOR THIS DISH IS "VICHY (*VEE-SHEE*) CARROTS," my kids call these "Vicious Carrots." A visiting friend once charmingly mispronounced the French name, and my daughters couldn't stop laughing. What could be less vicious than a carrot? Particularly in this seriously yummy recipe! Needless to say, the name stuck. Legend has it this recipe is adapted from a traditional French recipe that used Vichy mineral water. It's a great side dish with chicken. Be sure to use young, fresh carrots if you can find them—they'll be more tender.

> 2 tablespoons salted butter
>
> 1 tablespoon liquid honey (see Note)
>
> 12 young, fresh carrots, peeled and sliced into bite-size coins (about 2 cups)
>
> 1½ cups *Brodo* (page 301) or ready-to-use low-sodium vegetable broth
>
> 1 tablespoon chopped fresh flat-leaf parsley leaves
>
> Sea salt and ground black pepper, to taste

1. In a large skillet or wok over medium heat, melt the butter. Add the honey and stir vigorously for 1 minute, or until the mixture starts to bubble slightly. Add the carrots and stir to coat them well. Stir in the *brodo* (the carrots should be just covered). Bring the mixture to a boil, then reduce the heat to medium-high and simmer vigorously, uncovered, to allow the water to evaporate. (The dish should really be bubbling away!) Stir occasionally. After 15 to 20 minutes, the liquid will have reduced to a sauce (almost a glaze), and you'll have the most savory, melt-in-your-mouth carrots you've ever imagined eating. If it hasn't, pour off some of the liquid, turn up the heat slightly, and cook for a minute or two longer. Stir regularly (but gently) to make sure the carrots don't burn. Sprinkle with parsley, salt, and pepper, and serve immediately. *Bon appétit!*

Note: You can substitute an equal amount of sugar for the honey, if desired, but honey is better. Just remember that babies under 12 months aren't supposed to have unpasteurized honey.

Wow. The prep was so simple, and I can't say enough about the texture. You were right . . . it took cooked carrots to an entirely different level. —LORI

My 2-year-old ended up eating about five bites—for her that's positive feedback! They were delicious—very simple but a nice side dish. —TERESA

~~~~~~~~~~~~~~~~~~~~~

Ⓓ Grated Carrot Salad

10 minutes to prepare (10 minutes hands-on); serves 2 adults and 3 children

GRATED CARROT SALAD IS A FAVORITE DISH FOR FRENCH KIDS. THEY EAT IT regularly for school lunch, and it's popular at home as well. Even adults enjoy it as a starter.

The secret to this salad is in the texture: finely grated raw carrots that are simultaneously crisp and melt-in-your-mouth. The more finely grated the carrots, the more their natural sweetness comes out. For kids who have a hard time with crunchier textures, this might just be the dish that convinces them they love raw carrots. (You can also dress the salad with Classic Vinaigrette, page 302.)

> 8 large carrots
> ½ cup finely chopped fresh flat-leaf parsley leaves (do not use dried parsley)
> 2 tablespoons extra virgin olive oil
> Juice of 1 orange (about ½ cup)
> Juice of ½ lemon (about 1 tablespoon)
> Pinch sea salt
> ½ teaspoon Dijon mustard, optional
> Slices of lime, optional

1. Peel the carrots (important because the skin is often more bitter than the interior). Using a box grater or food processor fitted with the shredding blade, grate the carrots into fine shreds. (Food mills are popular in France and make fine, delicate shredded carrot—if you have one, use it!) Transfer the shredded carrots to a large bowl. Add the parsley and mix to combine.
2. Make the dressing: In a small bowl, combine the oil, orange and lemon juices, salt, and mustard, if using. Taste and add more oil or lemon juice, as desired.

3. Mix just enough dressing into the carrots to coat them lightly—do not overdress. Serve the salad at room temperature or slightly chilled (see Notes), topped with lime slices, if desired.

Notes: This salad is tasty when prepared fresh, but will be even more delicious if you let it marinate for a few hours, or even overnight, in the refrigerator. The parsley taste will mellow, and the sweetness of the carrots will be more intense.

For another great flavor combination, substitute Cilantro Lime Dressing: Combine ⅛ teaspoon freshly grated lime zest, 2 tablespoons fresh lime juice, 2 tablespoons finely chopped fresh cilantro leaves, and 2 tablespoons extra virgin olive oil. It's a fun way to introduce flavor variety after your children have got used to the standard carrot salad recipe.

I made the grated carrot salad with the cilantro lime dressing and the kids really enjoyed it. Will definitely make it again. Nice and fresh, and simple to make! —ROBERTA

The carrot salad was a big hit tonight. Lucas (3) dove right in and cleaned his plate! —JESSICA

CAULIFLOWER

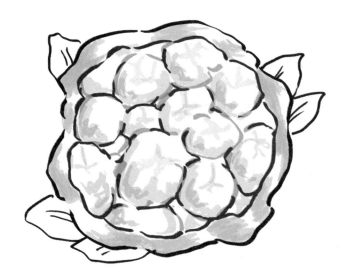

LOOKS JUST LIKE MASHED POTATOES!

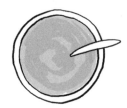

A YUMMY YELLOW PURÉE

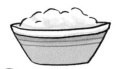

B MARVELOUS
MASHED CAULIFLOWER
(FAUX MASHED POTATOES)

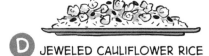

D JEWELED CAULIFLOWER RICE

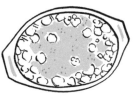

C CAULIFLOWER GRATIN

Yummy Yellow Purée

13 minutes to prepare (5 minutes hands-on); makes 4 to 6 baby jars

THE RICH YELLOW COLOR OF THIS RECIPE COMES FROM THE TURMERIC, A spice widely used in Asia and particularly in Indian cooking. Don't worry, turmeric is not spicy, but it still captures the warm, nutty essence of curry. It blends wonderfully with the cauliflower, giving it a subtle but interesting flavor.

Start by serving this dish to babies in small tasting portions: vegetables from the *Brassica* family (including cauliflower and broccoli) can give some people gassy tummies.

2 cups cauliflower florets
1 cup *Brodo* (page 301) or ready-to-use low-sodium vegetable broth
1 tablespoon salted butter
¼ teaspoon ground turmeric

1. Fill a medium saucepan with a few inches of water and bring to a boil over medium heat. Add the cauliflower and simmer for 7 to 8 minutes, or until the cauliflower is tender. Strain the cauliflower, reserving the cooking liquid.
2. In a blender, combine the cooked cauliflower, *brodo*, butter, and turmeric. Purée, adding enough cooking liquid to reach desired consistency.

Notes: Turmeric stains bright yellow! Cover the carpets when you're serving this dish to baby.

Here's a fun idea: choose one bib to use solely for foods that stain (such as beets and curry)—you can call it the curry bib.

Taste-Training Tip: If you want some of the traditional spice of a curry in this dish, try substituting ½ teaspoon curry powder for the turmeric. My younger adventurous eater loved it, and even the older, more cautious one warmed up.

B

Marvelous Mashed Cauliflower (Faux Mashed Potatoes)

25 minutes to prepare (5 minutes hands-on); serves 4 adults or 8 hungry children

MASHED OR CREAMED CAULIFLOWER IS A HEALTHY SUBSTITUTE FOR MASHED potatoes: fewer calories, more nutrients! But that's not what I tell my kids. I simply say, "It's yummy." Magically, they seem to agree.

I find most mashed cauliflower recipes too watery, but this recipe is creamy—just like "real" mashed potatoes. Quite a few of my test families were dubious—but they all loved it!

1 head cauliflower, chopped into bite-size pieces (about 6 cups)
½ clove garlic, optional
2 tablespoons buttermilk (see Note) or cream or milk (whatever you would normally use
   to make mashed potatoes)
2 tablespoons salted butter
Extra virgin olive oil, for garnish
Optional garnishes: ¼ cup chopped fresh cilantro, parsley, chives, or dill or cooked bacon

1. In a medium saucepan fitted with a steamer, bring 2 cups of water to a boil over high heat. Add the cauliflower and garlic, if using, and steam until very tender, 15 to 20 minutes. If you don't have a steamer, you can place the cauliflower and garlic in a microwave-safe bowl with ¼ cup of water, cover, and microwave on high for 5 minutes.
2. Transfer the cooked cauliflower and garlic to a food processor and add the buttermilk and butter. Process until just smooth (if you overprocess, it will get gooey). Serve hot, drizzled with olive oil and sprinkled with your garnish of choice.

Note: If you don't have buttermilk on hand, you can combine 2 tablespoons milk plus ¼ teaspoon lemon juice for similar results.

My daughter couldn't believe this wasn't mashed potatoes! She votes it as a total success of a recipe.
—JAMIE

I let the girls eat several bites, and then I told them it wasn't mashed potatoes. Before I told them, they wanted you to know your mashed potato recipe was "perfect" and "so yummy." I even served it with fried chicken and green beans, making the illusion complete. —LORI

I made this by mistake. I was planning to make the casserole but got busy helping my daughter with her homework and overcooked the cauliflower—so mashed it was! I loved it and had to hold myself back from eating it all. —ELENA

 ## Cauliflower Gratin

35 minutes to prepare (10 minutes hands-on); serves 2 adults and 2 older children

I LOVE THIS DISH, IN WHICH CAULIFLOWER IS BAKED IN A CLASSIC FRENCH béchamel (white) sauce. It's deceptively delicious: who would have thought such a great casserole could be produced from such simple flavors? (This recipe appeared in *French Kids Eat Everything* and was such a hit with readers that I've included it here.)

1 head cauliflower, chopped into bite-size pieces
   (about 6 cups)
3 tablespoons salted butter
3 tablespoons all-purpose flour
2 cups milk
Sea salt and ground black pepper, to taste
Pinch nutmeg, optional

Topping:
¼ cup dried breadcrumbs
¼ cup grated Parmesan cheese

1. Preheat the oven to 350°F and butter a baking dish.
2. Bring a medium saucepan of water to a boil over medium-high heat. Add the cauliflower and cook it at a rolling boil for 7 to 8 minutes, or until it's tender but slightly crunchy. Drain and set aside.
3. Meanwhile, make the white sauce: In a large skillet over medium heat, melt the butter. Sprinkle the flour into the butter and whisk until the flour is absorbed and forms a smooth paste. Immediately add the milk, whisking constantly (to avoid burning) until the sauce is the consistency of light cream, about 3 minutes. (Don't overcook it; it will continue to thicken in the oven.) Stir in the salt and pepper, and the nutmeg, if using. Set aside.

4. Make the topping: In a small bowl, combine the breadcrumbs and Parmesan.

5. Place the cooked cauliflower in the prepared baking dish. Pour the white sauce evenly overtop, sprinkle with the breadcrumb mixture, and bake in the oven for 15 minutes, or until the top is golden brown and crunchy. Prepare to be converted to a cauliflower lover!

I made this last night with my 22-month-old; it came out quite pretty—and delicious. She had fun helping me layer the veggies and sprinkle the breadcrumbs on top, and she was so eager to eat it that she didn't want to wait for it to bake! —ALICE

 ## Jeweled Cauliflower Rice

35 minutes to prepare (15 minutes hands-on); serves 2 adults and 2 toddlers

THIS DISH WAS INSPIRED BY A VISIT TO ONE OF MY FAVORITE VANCOUVER restaurants, Vij's, regularly voted one of the best Indian restaurants in North America. I had this dish only once, but I've been trying to recreate something like it ever since. This recipe has a few of my own twists (the addition of currants or raisins and the squeeze of fresh lime juice), and it isn't spicy like the adult version, but it will still please adult taste buds.

My kids love this dish, particularly the currants/raisins, which are soft, sweet, and slightly plump after being soaked in water. "They look like jewels," my younger daughter said once, and the name stuck. (Younger kids will have fun looking through their serving for their "jewels," but we have a rule: only one jewel per bite!)

1 teaspoon salted butter

1½ cups basmati rice (see Notes)

2 tablespoons vegetable oil

1 teaspoon cumin seeds

1 medium onion, chopped

5 whole cloves

½ teaspoon ground turmeric

1 head cauliflower, chopped into bite-size pieces (about 6 cups)

½ cup currants or raisins, soaked in ½ cup warm water

1 teaspoon sea salt, optional

¼ cup finely chopped fresh flat-leaf parsley or cilantro leaves

1 lime, optional

1. In a medium saucepan (with a lid) over medium-low heat, melt the butter. Add the rice, increase the heat to high, and cook, stirring vigorously, for 1 minute. Add 3 cups of water and bring to a boil; as soon as the water is boiling, cover the pan and reduce the heat to low. Simmer until the water is absorbed, 12 to 15 minutes. Turn off the heat but keep the lid on, and let the rice rest for 2 minutes. Uncover and set aside.

2. Meanwhile, in a skillet or wok over medium heat, heat the oil. Add the cumin seeds and let them sizzle in the pan for about 30 seconds, then add the onion and cloves. Sauté for 3 to 4 minutes, or until the onion is just starting to turn golden brown. Add the turmeric and sauté for 2 minutes, until the onion is well coated and the turmeric is absorbed. Add the cauliflower and currants with their soaking water, increase the heat to medium-high, and sauté for 5 minutes. Reduce the heat to medium-low, add salt, if using, cover, and cook for 5 minutes, or until the cauliflower is crisp-tender (cooked through but not too soft).

3. In a large bowl, combine the cooked rice, cauliflower mixture, and parsley and stir well. If desired, squeeze fresh lime juice overtop. Serve immediately (see Notes).

Notes: The key to pilaf is that each grain of rice should be fluffy and separate. The rice shouldn't be sticky. To achieve this, either soak the rice in warm water for 20 minutes (and then discard the water) or, using a fine-mesh strainer, rinse the rice under running water, rubbing it with your fingers to clean it. Either method will get rid of the starch that makes rice sticky.

Because rice can harbor bacteria that can cause food poisoning, this dish needs to be eaten immediately—no leftovers!

I made Jeweled Cauliflower Rice tonight. My 4-year-old was not too happy about it, saying it looked and smelled funny. Then she ate it and said, "It's delicious!" We couldn't get enough and even ran out.

—BABETTE

GREEN BEANS

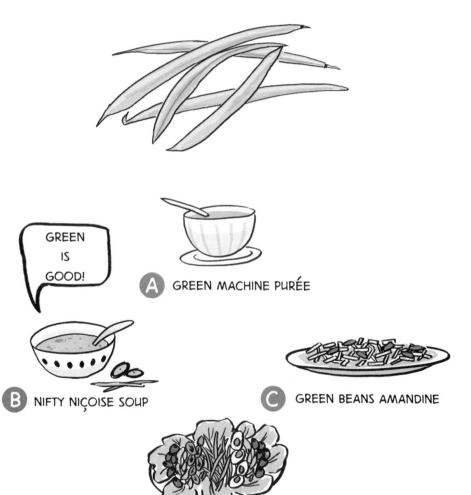

GREEN IS GOOD!

A GREEN MACHINE PURÉE

B NIFTY NIÇOISE SOUP

C GREEN BEANS AMANDINE

D SALAD NIÇOISE

Green Machine Purée

13 minutes to prepare (5 minutes hands-on); makes 6 to 8 baby jars

HAVE YOU EVER TASTED STORE-BOUGHT BABY "GREEN BEAN PURÉE"? IT'S bland, stodgy, and extremely boring. That's too bad, because green beans are actually quite tasty and packed full of nutrients. If *my* first impression of a green bean was the jarred purée . . . well, *yuck!* This recipe introduces kids and babies to a great-tasting version of a great-for-you food.

The garlic in this recipe is there for flavoring only (I often saw French parents using garlic to subtly flavor their baby purées). The secret is to cook the garlic with the other vegetables, but then remove it before making the purée. It will add a nice bit of flavor without the spicy bite.

I've suggested two methods below for cooking this dish: one fast (boiling the veggies) and one slow (simmering/steaming them). Slower cooking will retain more nutrients, but sometimes speed is of the essence.

> 3 cups water, *Brodo* (page 301), or ready-to-use low-sodium vegetable broth
> 1 cup trimmed and chopped green beans
> 1 small zucchini, cut into large chunks (1½ to 2 cups)
> ½ small clove garlic, optional
> 1 teaspoon dried basil or parsley

1. *Fast method (boiling):* Bring the water or *brodo* to a boil in a medium saucepan over medium-high heat. Add the beans, zucchini, and garlic, if using, and cook until the vegetables are tender, about 5 minutes. Reduce the heat to medium, add the basil, and simmer for 1 minute. Strain the vegetables, reserving the cooking liquid. Remove and discard the garlic. Transfer the vegetables with 1 cup of the cooking liquid to a blender or food processor and purée the vegetables, adding enough cooking liquid to reach desired consistency.

2. *Slower method (steaming):* In a medium saucepan fitted with a steamer insert, bring 2 cups of water to a boil over high heat. Add the garlic to the boiling water. In the steamer, layer the beans, then the zucchini, and steam until the vegetables are tender, about 15 minutes. Remove and discard the garlic and reserve the cooking

liquid. Transfer the vegetables to a blender or food processor and purée, slowly adding enough cooking liquid to reach desired consistency.

~~~~~~~~~~~~~~~~~~~~~

Ⓑ Nifty Niçoise Soup

20 minutes to prepare (5 minutes hands-on); serves 2 adults and 2 children (as a small "starter" soup)

THIS RECIPE USES THE FLAVOR PAIRING PRINCIPLE TO CREATE A MILD DISH that highlights the taste of green beans by pairing them with a hint of olives (an ingredient that brings out the flavor of the green beans). This anticipates the ingredients of Salad Niçoise (a healthy, tasty French classic that both kids and adults will love). Don't be deceived by the small quantities of some of the ingredients: they add a hint of flavor without overpowering the soup. Less is more in this case. (Some of my taste-testing adults found this recipe bland, but some of their kids preferred it that way.) This soup freezes well.

1 tablespoon olive oil

1 clove garlic, halved

2 carrots, peeled and cut into bite-size coins

1 cup green beans, trimmed and halved crosswise

3 cups *Brodo* (page 301) or ready-to-use low-sodium vegetable broth

2 cups chopped zucchini

2 green olives, pitted (see Note)

½ teaspoon dried basil

Topping (optional for older kids and adults):

¼ cup crumbled feta cheese

1 cup croutons

1. In a medium saucepan over medium heat, heat the oil for 1 minute. Add the garlic and sauté for 30 seconds, then add the carrots and green beans. Increase the heat to medium-high and cook for 3 minutes, stirring occasionally. Add the *brodo*, zucchini, and olives. Increase the heat to high, bring to a boil, and boil for 1 minute.

Reduce the heat to medium, add the basil, stirring to dissolve any clumps, and cook until the beans are very soft, 5 to 8 minutes. Remove from the heat. Using a blender, purée the soup.

Note: If you choose black olives instead, it's best to use high-quality ones from a trusted source, as chemicals are sometimes used to artificially turn olives black.

Taste-Training Tip: If your children don't like olives, have them try even a tiny nibble of an olive beforehand. This will prepare them for the slight taste of olives in this soup.

My 5-year-old was hesitant and didn't like the smell of this soup but took a bite. She said that it tasted "creamy," then ate most of it. When I told her it contained olives, she asked to taste a whole olive—which was new for her. My 2-year-old tasted the soup and said it tasted "like salad." She also wanted to try an olive and even enjoyed the pimento! —KRISTINE

I had the girls feel the olives beforehand. No one in my house (except me, of course) cares for green olives. I didn't tell them I was putting them in the soup, I just had them smell and feel them. They were certain: green olives look bad, smell bad, and surely taste bad. So when I poured the soup into the bowls, I was sure they wouldn't like it—but they did! No one could guess the aftertaste. I loved the looks on their faces when I told them it was green olives! —LORI

Baby Gabriel (8½ months old) wasn't crazy about it the first night, but ate it all up nights two and three! And the adults were big fans. —MIRA

 ## Green Beans Amandine

20 minutes to prepare (5 minutes hands-on); serves 2 adults and 2 children (at least)

THIS FRENCH DISH IS A MUCH-LOVED AMERICAN CLASSIC. MY VERSION OF the recipe lightens it up a bit (less fat, more crunch), but the essential flavors are still there. This is a great way to gussy up an old favorite—and a perfect match for that Sunday roast.

1 tablespoon salted butter

1 tablespoon olive oil

¾ cup sliced almonds

1½ pounds fresh green beans, trimmed and cut into bite-size pieces

Zest of ½ lemon

Sea salt and ground black pepper, to taste

1. Bring a large saucepan of water to a boil over high heat.

2. Meanwhile, in a large skillet over medium heat, melt the butter in the oil. Add the almonds and sauté for 3 to 4 minutes, stirring often, until the almonds start to smell like they're toasting. (Pay attention—they can burn quickly!) Remove the skillet from the heat and set aside.

3. When the water is boiling, add the green beans and reduce the heat to medium. Simmer the beans for 5 minutes, or until just tender. (Don't overcook or they'll be mushy.) Drain the beans, discarding the water.

4. Add the cooked beans to the skillet with the almonds and increase the heat to medium-high. Cook, stirring constantly, for about 1 minute, then add the lemon zest, salt, and pepper. Cook, stirring, for another 1 or 2 minutes to allow the flavors to mingle. (Optional: grate a little zest on top for added texture and color.) Serve immediately.

All three of my kids love green beans as well as almonds, so this was a hit. My 7-year-old said, "The beans are crunchy and so are the almonds!" My 5-year-old said, "I like both of them. They taste good together." And my 3-year-old said, "I'm eating all of it." And he did!

—ROBERTA

D Salad Niçoise

32 minutes to prepare (20 minutes hands-on); serves 2 adults and 2 children

I STARTED MAKING THIS DISH BECAUSE MY YOUNGER DAUGHTER WENT through an inconvenient phase where she didn't like eggs. Her older sister would eat them scrambled, hard-boiled, poached—you name it—but Claire had developed a bit of a mental block about them. So I made this salad with her, and she would pick out the things she liked. Gradually, ever so slowly, she'd begin trying bits of egg. Eventually she devoured them!

Traditionally, this classic French salad does not contain any cooked vegetables. It features raw vegetables, hard-boiled eggs, anchovies, olive oil, and, of course, niçoise olives. Lettuce, rice, and potatoes—ingredients made popular by Julia Child—aren't normally featured. Try it this way or add in your favorite ingredients—there are as many ways to make *salad niçoise* as there are chefs!

2 large eggs

2 cups green beans, trimmed and halved crosswise

½ head green lettuce (preferably romaine), torn into bite-size pieces

2 large ripe tomatoes, quartered

½ cup black niçoise olives, pitted

8 anchovy fillets, drained (if you buy them packed in oil) or 1 can tuna, drained

Dressing:

½ cup extra virgin olive oil

¼ cup red wine vinegar

¼ cup chopped fresh herbs (parsley and basil are best, but you can also use cilantro)

Sea salt and ground black pepper, to taste

½ clove garlic, minced, optional

1. Put the eggs in a small saucepan and pour in enough cold water to cover the eggs by 1 to 2 inches. Cover and bring the water to a boil over high heat. Once boiling, turn off the heat but leave the pan on the burner for 14 minutes—set your timer! (Cooking eggs this way keeps the shells from cracking, keeps the egg whites tender, and avoids that green-gray rim around the yolks.) Rinse the eggs under cold running water, then peel them and set aside.
2. Meanwhile, bring a medium saucepan of water to a rolling boil over high heat. Add the green beans, reduce the heat to medium-high, and cook for 7 to 8 minutes, or until just tender. Drain the beans and set aside.
3. Quarter the eggs or chop into small pieces.
4. Place the lettuce in the bottom of a large, preferably shallow, serving bowl. Arrange the tomatoes, cooked eggs, cooked beans, olives, and anchovies overtop.

5. Make the dressing: In a small bowl, whisk together the oil, vinegar, herbs, salt, pepper, and garlic, if using. Pour over the salad and serve immediately.

Taste-Training Tip: This is one of those dishes for which "combine your own" strategies sometimes works. On individual plates, lay out the lettuce together with the veggies that you know your child likes. Put the other ingredients in bowls on the table. Invite your child to add extra ingredients to make their own salad. Be sure you set the example of helping yourself to each bowl and enjoying the salad, too!

PEAS

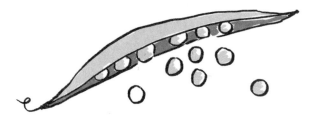

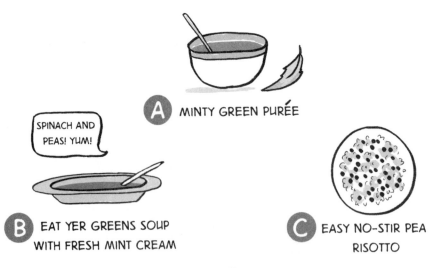

(A) MINTY GREEN PURÉE

SPINACH AND PEAS! YUM!

(B) EAT YER GREENS SOUP WITH FRESH MINT CREAM

(C) EASY NO-STIR PEA RISOTTO

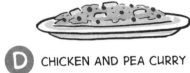

(D) CHICKEN AND PEA CURRY

Minty Green Purée

10 minutes to prepare (2 minutes hands-on); makes about 2 cups or 4 to 6 baby jars

PEA PURÉE IS A POPULAR SIDE DISH IN BRITAIN, WHERE IT'S MASHED, flavored with mint, and served alongside lamb. This version uses just a small amount of mint to gently introduce the taste, and adds zucchini to lighten the texture of the purée, which makes it smooth and creamy. For an extra-creamy taste, you can add yogurt, sour cream, milk, or any dairy substitute.

10- or 12-ounce package frozen peas, thawed
1 large or two medium potatoes, peeled and chopped
3 to 4 fresh mint leaves
1 medium zucchini, peeled and chopped
2 tablespoons Greek yogurt, sour cream, or milk, optional
1 tablespoon salted butter
Pinch sea salt

1. Bring 4 cups of water to a rolling boil in a medium saucepan over high heat. Add the peas, potatoes, and mint and return to a boil. Reduce the heat to medium-high and simmer for 5 minutes. Add the zucchini and cook for 3 minutes, until the potatoes are cooked through. Strain the vegetables, reserving the cooking liquid.
2. In the same pan, combine the cooked vegetables with 1 cup of the cooking liquid. Using a food processor or immersion blender, purée until smooth. For a creamier purée, mix in the yogurt, if using. Stir in the butter and salt. If needed, add more cooking liquid to reach desired consistency. For a very fine purée, push the mixture through a fine-mesh sieve before serving. Serve warm.

Taste-Testing Tip: This is a great recipe to use if you would like to introduce the taste of fish to babies (some pediatricians recommend introducing fish at 9 months, others at 12 months). Simply add 2 ounces of fresh white fish (such as sole) when you cook the peas, first making sure there are no fish bones, and purée as directed. *Voilà!*

Ⓑ Eat Yer Greens Soup with Fresh Mint Cream

25 minutes to prepare (5 minutes hands-on); serves 2 adults and 2 children

PEAS ARE RICH IN MINERALS, VITAMINS, AND FIBER, AND THEY TASTE good—slightly sweet and quite flavorful. If you introduce them to kids early, most will learn to love them. Plus, peas are a great base from which to springboard to more adventurous taste training. Once your child has learned to love peas, you can start adding other tastes. This recipe combines the flavors of the Minty Green Purée (page 207) and Sophie's Spinach Surprise (page 221) for a lovely soup that the whole family can eat together.

This soup freezes well, but make the Fresh Mint Cream just before serving.

3 tablespoons salted butter

1 medium onion, chopped

½ teaspoon mild curry powder (see Notes)

One 10-ounce package frozen peas, thawed

One 10-ounce package frozen chopped spinach, thawed (or 2 cups fresh)

3 cups *Brodo* (page 301) or ready-to-use low-sodium vegetable or chicken broth

½ cup fresh mint leaves, chopped

1 cup milk (see Notes)

½ teaspoon ground black pepper

½ teaspoon sea salt, optional

Fresh Mint Cream:

¼ cup fresh mint leaves, chopped

½ cup crème fraîche

1. In a large saucepan over medium heat, melt the butter. Add the onion and curry powder, stirring well, and sauté until the onion starts to turn golden, 4 to 5 minutes.

2. Add the peas, spinach, and *brodo*. Bring the mixture to a boil, then reduce the heat to medium-low and simmer for 5 minutes. Add the ½ cup mint and simmer for 5 minutes, or until the peas are tender.

3. Meanwhile, make the Fresh Mint Cream: In a blender, combine the ¼ cup mint and crème fraîche and purée until smooth. Set aside.

4. Remove the soup from the heat and stir in the milk and pepper, and the salt, if using.

Transfer the mixture to a blender or food processor and purée until completely smooth. Serve immediately, topped with the mint cream. (I sometimes make little happy faces for the kids—one drop for each eye, a dollop for the nose, a curly swirl for the mouth—but they love to make up their own designs, too.)

Notes: For more tentative kids, omit the curry powder. As their tastes change, you can introduce it, eventually increasing the amount of curry powder to 1 teaspoon or more.

If needed, you can use a milk substitute; it will, however, change the texture considerably.

Blended soups, particularly with additions of things like mint, are completely new to my culinary repertoire, so I'm happy to discover them. Francesca, age 4, was very excited to make smiley faces in her soup. She said, "It smells like garlic. I like it!" —MIRA

Easy No-Stir Pea Risotto

35 minutes to prepare (5 minutes hands-on); serves 2 adults and 3 children (as a main course with generous servings)

THIS DISH WAS ONE OF THE TOP FIVE FAVORITES AMONG ALL MY TEST FAMI-lies. The kids at the Alphabet Academy gave it an enthusiastic thumbs up: 15 out of 17 preschoolers loved it and wanted more!

It's funny, because this dish almost didn't make it into the book. Given my absent-mindedness—my husband christened me *"La Reine des Casseroles Brûlés"* (Queen of Burned Pots) soon after we were married—I was terrified of making risotto until an Italian friend of mine showed me this oven-baked version that doesn't require you to stir, and stir, and stir—magic! The texture is a bit different from that of the stovetop version—a tiny bit less creamy—but it's still delicious.

5 cups *Brodo* (page 301) or ready-to-use low-sodium vegetable or chicken broth

1½ cups risotto rice (see Notes)

1 cup grated Parmesan cheese

3 tablespoons salted butter

½ teaspoon sea salt, optional (see Notes)

1 teaspoon ground black pepper

1 cup frozen peas, thawed

1 teaspoon fresh lemon juice, optional

1. Preheat the oven to 350°F. In a medium saucepan over medium-low heat, bring the *brodo* to a simmer.
2. In a Dutch oven or large baking dish, combine the rice and 4 cups of the hot *brodo*. Cover (use foil, if necessary) and bake in the oven for 30 minutes, until most of the liquid is absorbed and the rice is just slightly firm to the bite (al dente).
3. Remove the dish from the oven and stir in the Parmesan, remaining 1 cup of hot *brodo*, butter, salt, if using, and pepper. Stir vigorously until the rice is thick and creamy, 2 to 3 minutes. Add the peas and stir until heated through. Add the lemon juice, if using. Serve immediately (the risotto tends to get thicker and stodgier if you wait).

Notes: I prefer to use Carnaroli or Arborio rice for this dish. Some readers have reported success using brown rice—if that is all you have, give it a go!

Parmesan cheese is salty, so I would not add too much salt to this dish—salt it at the table if necessary.

Because rice can harbor bacteria that can cause food poisoning, this dish needs to be eaten immediately and not used for leftovers. Plus, the texture will get mushy.

Very easy to make and incredibly tasty! My wife thought this was great comfort food and in the same class as high-quality macaroni and cheese made from scratch. —Jon

I just can't get enough of this recipe. It's too easy for such buttery-risotto results! The girls were lukewarm about it on the first try, and on the second attempt—in which it was essentially the same—they cleaned their bowls and asked why hadn't I made this before. "So delicious!" Kids are funny. —Lori

Today we served the Easy No-Stir Pea Risotto to our preschool classes. The children enjoyed the rice and commented that it was nice and soft but not squishy. We heard quite a bit of "it tastes like pasta with cheese" and that "the peas are sweet." One child commented, "She put yummies in there!" —Alphabet Academy

(D) Chicken and Pea Curry

30 minutes to prepare (10 minutes hands-on); serves 2 adults and 2 children (as a main course)

THANKS TO THE EASY NO-STIR PEA RISOTTO (PAGE 209) AND EAT YER Greens Soup with Fresh Mint Cream (page 208) recipes, your child is now familiar with the texture of peas and rice, as well as with the taste of turmeric—a key ingredient in curry. Time for the big leagues! This very mild curry is a great way to introduce your child to the taste of Indian food. I serve this curry with rice and mango chutney. *Yum!*

In my family, we experiment with this recipe: sometimes I'll add thinly sliced carrot, or a garlic clove; other times I leave out the sweet potato. The possibilities are endless! But do make sure to try this recipe with the apple—the sweetness offsets the curry, and the melt-in-your-mouth texture of the cooked apple is a nice complement to the chicken.

1 tablespoon vegetable oil

1 tablespoon mild curry paste (see Notes)

1 tablespoon tomato paste

1 medium sweet potato, peeled and cut into bite-size pieces

1 carrot, peeled and diced

1 large apple, peeled, cored, and thinly sliced

2 large boneless, skinless chicken breasts, cut into bite-size pieces

One 14-ounce can coconut milk

1 cup *Brodo* (page 301) or ready-to-use low-sodium vegetable or chicken broth

One 10-ounce package frozen peas (or equivalent fresh)

½ cup chopped fresh cilantro, for garnish

Cooked rice, for serving

Mango chutney, for serving

1. In a wok or deep skillet over high heat, heat the oil. Stir in the curry paste, reduce heat, and gently cook for 1 minute. Stir in the tomato paste. Add sweet potato, carrot, apple, and chicken, stirring until well coated. Cook, stirring often, for 5 minutes. Pour in the coconut milk and *brodo*. Increase the heat to high and bring to a boil. Once boiling, immediately reduce the heat to medium and simmer for 5 minutes. Add the peas and simmer for 5 minutes more, until the peas are tender (but not mushy). Serve over cooked rice with mango chutney on the side. *Delish!*

Notes: I like to use korma curry paste in this recipe. Adventurous eaters may want to increase the amount used to 2 tablespoons.

If you feel this dish needs salt, just sprinkle a tiny pinch of salt on each dish before serving. You'll taste the salt more, but will actually be eating less.

The spice level was perfect for the kids, and they really enjoyed it. My boys' comments: my 7-year-old said, "Good! But maybe add some cashews to it the next time" (I kid you not); my 5-year-old said, "I like that it's kind of sugary" (he's referring to the sweetness of the apples); and my 3-year-old said, "I like the peas and the chicken." I thought it was great and will definitely make it again. —ROBERTA

PEPPERS

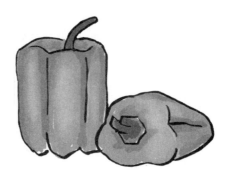

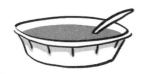

HOW DEEP
CAN YOU DIP IN?

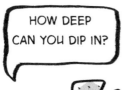

A ROASTED RED PEPPER
AND TOMATO SOUP

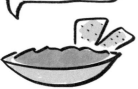

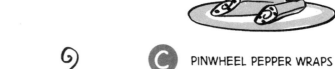

B RED ROCKET HUMMUS

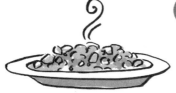

C PINWHEEL PEPPER WRAPS

D RATATOUILLE
(SOUTHERN FRENCH STEW)

Roasted Red Pepper and Tomato Soup

20 minutes to prepare (5 minutes hands-on); serves 2 adults and 2 children

I KNOW, I KNOW, ROASTING AND PEELING RED PEPPERS SOUNDS A LITTLE time-consuming. Let me reassure you: I have tried this recipe with both store-bought and fresh, do-it-yourself roasted red peppers, and the soup made with the store-bought kind is just as good. (Of course, if you want to roast them yourself, be my guest!)

Some adult versions of this recipe use sugar and chicken broth, but I prefer to use the juice of one orange and vegetable broth—the soup is naturally sweet, and the tomato and pepper flavors are complemented, but not overpowered, by the broth.

This soup freezes well.

1 tablespoon olive oil
¼ onion, chopped
½ small garlic clove (see Note)
5 large ripe tomatoes, cored and quartered
2 large or 3 small roasted red bell peppers
¼ cup chopped fresh basil leaves
4 cups *Brodo* (page 302) or ready-to-use low-sodium vegetable broth
Juice of 1 orange (about ½ cup)
Parmesan cheese, thinly sliced, optional
Fresh basil leaves, for garnish, optional

1. In a large saucepan over medium heat, heat the oil. Add the onion and garlic and sauté until the onion is translucent, about 3 minutes. Increase the heat to high and add the tomatoes, red peppers, and basil. Cook, stirring constantly, for 1 minute. Stir in the *brodo,* then reduce the heat to medium and simmer for 10 minutes. Stir in the orange juice. Using a blender, purée the soup until creamy smooth. Serve immediately, topped with Parmesan and a basil leaf, if desired (the cheese will melt into the soup, making it more creamy).

Note: I don't chop the garlic because small pieces can burn. The garlic will get puréed at the end anyway.

Adult Serving Tip: This soup is delicious, hot or cold, garnished with croutons. Stirring a bit of basil or cilantro pesto into this soup makes it divine! Also try serving this with a black olive tapenade on the side.

This soup was great. Kids loved it, husband loved it. I put crackers on the side. I didn't get many comments; that's what I noticed happens when they like it—they just eat it up! —FRANÇOISE

We had this soup for lunch today with some Cheddar cheese shredded on top and it was an absolute hit! Surprising, since they're not big fans of puréed soups, but all three kids loved it. My oldest called it "pizza soup" because he thought it tasted like pizza. Definitely something I will be making again. —ROBERTA

Red Rocket Hummus

20 minutes to prepare (10 minutes hands-on); serves 2 adults and 2 children or makes about 12 baby jars

THIS RECIPE USES CREAM (YES, I SAID CREAM). IT OFFSETS THE ACIDITY OF the peppers and tomatoes while enhancing their flavor (the French are never afraid of using a little fat). If you prefer, you can substitute yogurt.

For older babies, you can add 1 stalk of fennel, a bay leaf, and ½ clove garlic to gently flavor the soup (but make sure you remove them before you purée it).

Like most of the purée recipes in this book, this makes a lovely dish for adults—it's really a red pepper hummus in disguise.

This hummus freezes well.

½ clove garlic, optional (see Notes)
1 ripe tomato, quartered
1 red bell pepper, cored, seeded, and sliced
One 14-ounce can chickpeas, rinsed and drained
1 tablespoon whipping (35%) cream (see Notes)
1 tablespoon extra virgin olive oil
Juice of ½ lemon (about 1 tablespoon)
Pinch sea salt, optional

1. In a medium saucepan fitted with a steamer insert, bring 3 cups of water to a boil over medium heat. Add the garlic, if using, to the water. In the steamer, cook the tomato and red pepper for 7 to 8 minutes, or until the red pepper is tender. Strain the tomato and pepper, reserving the cooking liquid and discarding the garlic.
2. In a food processor, combine the cooked tomato and red pepper with the chickpeas, cream, oil, and lemon juice and purée until smooth. If too thick, slowly add enough cooking liquid to reach desired consistency. (Adults may want to add the salt to their serving.)

Notes: As your child grows, you can increase the intensity of the garlic in the recipe. For younger babies, boil the garlic in the water while you're steaming the tomato and pepper, then discard the garlic, as described in the recipe; the hummus will have just a hint of garlic flavor. For older kids, rather than discarding the cooked garlic, include it in the purée. This will lend a nice flavor to the hummus and is a lovely introduction to garlic.

If desired, you can substitute an equal amount of full-fat yogurt for the cream. For babies over 12 months, try substituting 1 tablespoon light tahini.

Pinwheel Pepper Wraps

5 minutes to prepare (5 minutes hands-on); serves 2 adults and 2 children

REMEMBER HOW POPULAR PINWHEEL WRAPS WERE IN THE 1990S? WELL, IT turns out that kids still like them. This simple recipe combines the crunchy texture of fresh red pepper with a smooth, savory cream cheese filling. These are great for school lunches. They're also a good recipe on which to test out your marketing tactics. The color swirls look fun; ask your kids to come up with interesting names.

It really helps to warm the tortillas first: warm, fresh tortillas bring out the flavors of the other ingredients, and they are much easier to chew than those at room temperature.

4 small flour tortillas
4 tablespoons cream cheese or Red Rocket Hummus (page 215)
1 small red bell pepper, cored, seeded, and finely chopped

Optional fillings (as your child grows older):

Avocado slices

Cooked sliced chicken

Roasted red pepper spread

Chopped fresh basil leaves

1. In a dry skillet over medium-low heat, gently warm the tortillas on each side. Transfer the tortillas to a clean work surface and spread 1 tablespoon cream cheese on top of each tortilla, then sprinkle each evenly with 1 tablespoon red pepper. Fold the sides and bottom of each tortilla up over the filling, then roll tightly to close. Using a sharp knife, slice the rolls diagonally into ½-inch-thick slices and serve immediately.

Note: Some smaller children may have trouble chewing these. You can cut the pinwheels into little pieces so they can eat them with a fork (or fingers).

We tried the pinwheels tonight. Über-cautious 3-year-old Lucas took one look at it and said, "I wonder what this tastes like?" and then popped it in his mouth! I was shocked! He didn't love them, but he did have a few bites. And he was very interested in how they looked. We will be trying them again for sure. —JESSICA

The children in our classrooms were very eager to see what was going to be served today. The votes are in: out of 40, 34 would like to have it on our menu. We recorded a lot of "crunchy," "sweet," "yummy, I want more!" and "great mix of crunchy and chewy!" We also heard, "I've never liked peppers, but now I like them—they are so delicious." Our favorite: "Mmmm, I tasted it with my taste bugs!" —ALPHABET ACADEMY

Ratatouille (Southern French Stew)

35 minutes to prepare (10 minutes hands-on); serves 2 adults and 2 children (as a main dish)

RATATOUILLE (*RA-TA-TOO-EE*) IS TRADITIONALLY A SUMMER DISH (THE vegetables called for all ripen in late summer), but it's one of my children's favorite dishes at any time of the year.

There are many ways to make ratatouille, but they basically divide into two approaches. The "slow food" approach insists that each vegetable needs to be peeled, then sautéed individually, and then the entire dish slowly roasted for hours. I've had it made this way—and it is indeed totally delicious—but it's also unrealistically time-consuming. The "grandmother's stew" approach (my preference) insists that this was always a simple dish that was left to simmer on the stove for hours, with no fuss. This is the way I make it, as a more liquid dish with a yummy broth that kids love. You don't need to peel the veggies (but you may if you like).

We also use ratatouille as a pasta sauce (you might want to simmer it for a bit longer, to thicken it up a bit more), eat it with roast chicken, and even use it as an ingredient in quiche. Or you can add chicken broth and blend it as a soup (remove the bay leaves first!), which freezes really well.

3 tablespoons olive oil

2 large leeks, white and green parts, finely sliced

2 teaspoons sea salt

1 medium eggplant, peeled and cut into ½-inch chunks

1 clove garlic, halved

1 red bell pepper, cored, seeded, and cut into big chunks

8 to 10 large ripe tomatoes, cored and quartered

1 large zucchini, peeled and cut into ½-inch chunks

1 tablespoon herbes de Provence (usually includes rosemary, thyme, basil, marjoram)

2 bay leaves

1 generous tablespoon liquid honey, packed dark brown sugar, or pure maple syrup

½ teaspoon ground black pepper

½ cup finely chopped fresh flat-leaf parsley leaves

1. In a large saucepan over medium-low heat, heat the oil. Add the leek and ½ teaspoon salt and sauté for about 5 minutes, or until the leeks are just starting to turn golden. Add the eggplant and garlic and stir well; cover and sauté for another 5 minutes, or until the eggplant is tender. Add the red pepper, tomatoes, zucchini, herbs, bay leaves, honey, remaining 1½ teaspoons salt, pepper, and parsley. Cover, increase the heat to high, bring to a near-boil, then reduce the heat to medium, cover, and cook, stirring occasionally, until all of the vegetables are perfectly tender, 10 to 15 minutes. Discard the bay leaves. Serve warm.

Time-Saving Tip: This dish comes together quickly because it cooks in stages: while one veggie is sautéing, you can chop the next one.

Note: This dish tastes great when first cooked, but is even better after it has sat for a few hours, once the flavors have melded. I try to make it the night before, cool it, and refrigerate it overnight. When reheated, the flavors become more savory. The restaurant La Note in Berkeley, California, serves ratatouille on a bed of couscous, topped with poached eggs; this transforms it from a side dish into a main course.

I thought this dish had great layering of flavor and was just yummy. I served it with orecchiette, my favorite pasta, and it was my favorite meal of the week. The kids took seconds, along with everyone at the table. There were no leftovers! —LORI

SPINACH

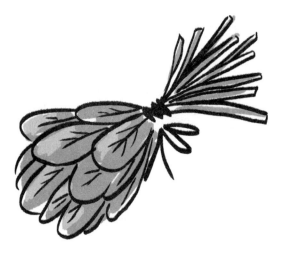

B SOPHIE'S SPINACH SURPRISE

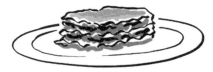
C SPEEDY SALMON SPINACH
LASAGNA

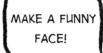
MAKE A FUNNY
FACE!

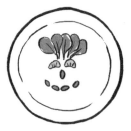
D WARM SPINACH
CITRUS SALAD

Sophie's Spinach Surprise

7 minutes to prepare (2 minutes hands-on); makes 4 to 6 baby jars

THIS RECIPE APPEARED IN *FRENCH KIDS EAT EVERYTHING*, AS IT WAS ONE of the first dishes I made to encourage our daughters to eat more vegetables. It worked like a charm! Several years later—even though they both eventually graduated to other green vegetables—my kids still love this dish (which I now serve as a starter soup in small ramekins).

This dish is mild and incredibly smooth and is an easy way to introduce your children to green vegetables. The zucchini provides a light, almost fluffy, melt-in-your-mouth texture, so that the spinach tastes airy and almost sweet. If you think the dish is still bitter (although I never do), add a tiny bit of honey before serving (or use a little less spinach).

This dish freezes wonderfully well and reheats quickly. But you may want to add a little water when reheating, as it tends to thicken slightly after being frozen.

> 1 medium or large zucchini, peeled and chopped (about 2 cups)
>
> 2 or 3 big handfuls baby spinach leaves (about 1 cup, tightly packed)
>
> 1 teaspoon salted butter, optional
>
> Whipping (35%) cream, optional
>
> Pinch sea salt, optional

1. In a medium saucepan over high heat, combine the zucchini and 1 cup of water. Bring to a boil, reduce the heat to medium, and simmer until the zucchini becomes transparent, about 2 minutes. Stir in the spinach and cook for 1 or 2 minutes, just until the spinach wilts. (Don't overcook the spinach or it will become slimy.) Strain the vegetables, reserving the cooking liquid. Remove the pan from the heat and, using a blender, purée until perfectly smooth, adding enough cooking liquid to reach desired consistency. Stir in butter, cream, and salt, if desired.

Taste-Training Tips: I've served spinach to both of my children for years, without any issues—spinach is one of their favorite foods!—however, because of its potentially high nitrate content, you should avoid serving spinach to babies younger than 12 months old and limit the amount you serve at any one sitting. Serve the purée in a small bowl as a side dish rather than as the main meal (I find that a little goes a long way.) Top it with tiny dabs of butter in the form of a happy face—your child will love to watch them melt. Encourage your child to "catch" the eyes (or nose or mouth) before they disappear.

Older kids and adults will enjoy this with the optional cream, butter, and salt, but little ones will eat this plain and love it, so serve it to them plain first.

Speedy Salmon Spinach Lasagna

1 hour to prepare (20 minutes hands-on); serves 4 adults and 2 children with generous servings

THIS IS A RECIPE THE WHOLE FAMILY WILL ENJOY, AND IT'S ONE OF THE dishes I love serving to guests, particularly out-of-town visitors, for whom I'll use fresh salmon (one of Vancouver's local delicacies) when it's in season. The salmon becomes very tender as it bakes in the béchamel sauce and is offset by the smooth firmness of the ricotta-spinach layers. Both of my daughters liked this lasagna as toddlers.

This recipe works just as well with canned salmon (in fact, some members of my family think it's even better). In recognition that good, fresh ingredients are sometimes hard to find, I've included frozen and canned options for this recipe—that's what makes it speedy!

3 tablespoons salted butter

3 tablespoons all-purpose flour

3 cups milk

One 6- to 7.5-ounce can wild salmon, larger bones and skin removed

1 tablespoon dried oregano

1 teaspoon sea salt, optional

1 teaspoon ground black pepper, optional

One 16-ounce container ricotta cheese

One 10-ounce package thawed and drained frozen spinach or 1 small bunch fresh
    spinach, cut into ½-inch pieces

2 large eggs

1 teaspoon ground cinnamon

9 to 12 fresh or cooked lasagna noodles (see Note)

2 cups shredded Cheddar cheese

½ cup grated Parmesan cheese

¼ cup chopped capers, for garnish, optional

1. Preheat the oven to 375°F.

2. Make the salmon béchamel sauce: In a medium saucepan over high heat, melt the butter. Add the flour and cook, whisking constantly, for 1 minute, until a smooth paste forms. Whisk in the milk and cook for 1 minute, or until the paste dissolves. Reduce the heat to medium and cook, stirring constantly, until the sauce begins to thicken, 3 to 4 minutes. Add the salmon, stirring well to break up the chunks, and oregano, and the salt and pepper, if using. Set aside.

3. In a large bowl, stir together the ricotta, spinach, eggs, and cinnamon.

4. In a baking dish, assemble the lasagna by layering the ingredients in the following order (as you make the layers, be sure the lasagna noodles are in contact with the béchamel sauce everywhere—if they don't absorb the sauce, they'll stay hard):

   Half the salmon béchamel sauce
   1 layer lasagna noodles
   All the spinach-ricotta filling
   1 layer lasagna noodles
   All but ¼ cup remaining salmon béchamel sauce (reserve some for the top)
   1 layer lasagna noodles

5. Drizzle the top of the lasagna with the reserved ¼ cup salmon béchamel sauce. Sprinkle evenly with the Cheddar, Parmesan, and, if using, capers (the capers add a bit of zing for older kids and adults). Bake in the oven for 30 minutes, or until the topping is golden and crunchy and the filling is bubbling. Set aside to cool for at least 10 minutes before serving (the filling will be piping hot straight out of the oven; cooled slightly, the lasagna will be much firmer and hold its shape better when sliced, as the ricotta filling helps the pieces hold their shape).

Note: You'll need enough lasagna noodles to create 3 layers, using 3 to 4 noodles per layer.

Serving Tip: This is a mild, almost delicate lasagna. Try serving it after a fresh starter salad with a tangy vinaigrette; the tastes will complement one another nicely. For a nice garnish, sprinkle a bit of dried oregano or parsley on top.

I made the Speedy Salmon Spinach Lasagna tonight. Wow, what a surprise. I had no idea what to expect from these combinations (very un-Midwestern indeed!), but you were right: it came together very easily and set up and cut beautifully. I'm very happy with this recipe. It was elegant and unique. Sara cleaned her plate, and even my picky eater Kelly ate half. Thanks for once again opening my mind and my palate! —LORI

To be honest, I was worried about this one. It sounded like an odd combo, and my kids are used to more traditional lasagna. My first pleasant surprise was the canned salmon. I have never used it before. It was great and not at all fishy! The lasagna was really interesting. It looked beautiful and cut nicely. My 7-year-old (my pickiest eater) did the best with it. On a scale of 1 to 10, he gave it a "150." —STACY

This was easy and deliciously creamy. My 3-year-old liked it and ate it all. His only comment was "good." My 5- and 7-year-olds liked the salt and chopped capers. —ROBERTA

I was a little worried the flavor was going to be boring, but it was delicious. I liked it because it wasn't overly rich despite the béchamel, and I felt super healthy with all the salmon and spinach. There's still some left over in the freezer, so it made three meals for the three of us. Love it! My 2-year-old didn't touch it at dinner (we're having power struggles right now) and went to bed hungry, but then inhaled the leftovers at lunch the next day. —TERESA

(D) Warm Spinach Citrus Salad

7 minutes to prepare (5 minutes hands-on); serves 2 adults and 2 children (small servings)

MY KIDS NOW LOVE LETTUCE AND SPINACH. BUT I ADMIT THAT IT TOOK A while. We started off with a toddler version of this salad, in which I served the ingredients as a happy face on a plate (5 or 6 spinach leaves for hair, mandarin orange pieces for eyes, half a cherry tomato for a nose, and so on). These happy faces take only a minute to make (as you pluck the pieces out of the salad you've made for the adults), and the kids can even help make them when they are older. The kids would dip their pieces in homemade vinaigrette, getting used to the taste and texture of salad, which we served first, before the main course. Eventually they proudly graduated to "grown-up" salad (although I admit to still surprising my younger one, now in kindergarten, with a salad happy face once in a while).

If you're starting the process with toddlers, remember that the happy face version isn't necessarily about your children eating a lot of salad. It's about them learning to *like the idea* of eating salad. Most kids won't start eating larger quantities until they're older.

4 cups loosely packed baby spinach (see Note)

2 mandarin oranges or clementines, peeled and separated into segments

½ cup cherry tomatoes, halved

¼ cup Classic Vinaigrette (page 302)

1. Heat a medium saucepan over medium heat. Wash the spinach under cool running water, then immediately place it in the pan and toss as you would a salad. As soon as you hear a hissing sound (which means that the water is evaporating off the spinach), remove the pan from the heat. The spinach should be slightly (*just* slightly) wilted.

2. In a medium bowl, combine three-quarters of both the oranges and tomatoes. Add the cooked spinach, then top with the remaining oranges and tomatoes. Don't toss the salad or the spinach will lose volume. Serve immediately with the vinaigrette on the side. (You can serve the vinaigrette mixed in as well, but be sure not to overtoss the salad.)

Note: Baby spinach leaves are smaller and quite tender compared with regular spinach leaves. They are wonderful combined with the slightly acidic oranges and tomatoes, and the vitamin C in the citrus and tomatoes helps you absorb the iron in the spinach.

I decided to make the salad, as my kids have a phobia about salads. I realized that making the happy face is still worth it for 6- and 9-year-olds—they loved it! And warming up the spinach made all the difference; they liked the soft texture. —FRANÇOISE

SQUASH

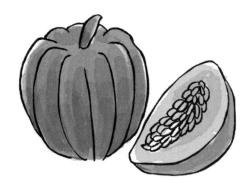

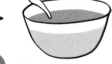

A SQUISH SQUASH SOUP

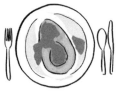

B ROAST SQUASH WITH
MAPLE DRESSING

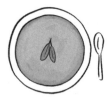

C SQUASH SAGE SOUP

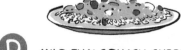

D MILD THAI SQUASH CURRY

Squish Squash

55 minutes to prepare (10 minutes hands-on); makes 2 to 3 cups or 4 to 6 baby jars (depending how big your squash is)

THIS PURÉE TAKES A LITTLE LONGER TO PREPARE THAN MOST OF THE OTHER recipes in the book, but it has two great advantages: it makes a delicious adult side dish (I've provided quantities based on the assumption that adults will eat it, too) and the recipe's funny name might persuade reluctant eaters to try a bite or two!

1 large butternut squash
1 tablespoon salted butter or vegetable oil
2 ripe pears or apples, peeled, cored, and quartered
Pinch sea salt, optional
½ teaspoon ground cinnamon, optional
Zest of ½ orange, optional

1. Preheat the oven to 400°F.
2. Halve the squash lengthwise and remove the seeds and stringy pulp. Rub the insides with butter. Place squash, cut-side down, in a baking dish with ¼ cup of water. Bake in the oven for 30 minutes, then add the pears. Bake for another 15 to 20 minutes, or until the squash is tender when pricked with a fork.
3. Remove the dish from the oven and set aside to cool slightly, at least 3 to 5 minutes. Using a spoon, scoop out the flesh from the cooked squash and transfer it to a blender or food processor. Add the cooked pears and purée until smooth. For younger babies, add enough water to reach desired consistency. For older children and adults, add salt, cinnamon, and orange zest, if desired.

Time-Saving Tip: This recipe can be made in half the time by boiling rather than baking the squash and pears. Simply cook the peeled, cubed butternut squash in boiling water until tender. Add the pears in the last few minutes of cooking or they'll dissolve into the water.

Ⓑ Roasted Squash with Maple Dressing

45 minutes to prepare (5 minutes hands-on); serves 2 adults and 2 children

THIS IS A GREAT DISH TO MAKE FOR BABIES WHO ARE TRANSITIONING TO more solid foods but who aren't really ready to chew hard foods or chunks. My younger daughter (who took a long, long time to start chewing solid foods) loved this dish, and we still make it on winter nights.

The taste-training element is in the dressing: the sweetness of the maple syrup and the acidity of the orange offsets the sage leaves, which pairs wonderfully with the squash.

Maple Dressing:
¼ cup pure maple syrup
¼ cup orange juice
¼ teaspoon ground cinnamon
4 fresh sage leaves

1 large butternut squash
1 tablespoon salted butter or vegetable oil
1 teaspoon sea salt, optional

1. Preheat the oven to 400°F.
2. Halve the squash lengthwise and remove the seeds and stringy pulp. Rub the insides with butter. Place squash, cut-side down, in a baking dish with ¼ cup of water. Bake in the oven for 30 to 40 minutes, or until tender when pricked with a fork. Remove from the oven, sprinkle with salt, if using, and set aside to cool.
3. Meanwhile, make the Maple Dressing: In a small saucepan over medium-low heat, combine the maple syrup, orange juice, and cinnamon and heat it gently for about 5 minutes. (*Bonus: this will make your kitchen smell wonderful!*) Set aside.
4. Make the crispy sage leaves: In the same skillet over medium heat, melt the remaining butter. Add the whole sage leaves and sauté until they are browned and slightly curled at the edges, about 3 minutes. Transfer the crispy sage leaves to a plate lined with paper towel (to absorb excess butter) and set aside.
5. Using a spoon, scoop out the flesh from the cooked squash and transfer it to a blender. Add the maple mixture and blend until smooth and creamy. Alternatively, for older

kids and adults, you can serve the squash halves whole, with the maple cinnamon sauce served in a little bowl on the side so kids can drizzle it in themselves.

6. Serve warm, topped with crispy sage leaves.

 ## Squash Sage Soup

1 hour to prepare (10 minutes hands-on); serves 2 adults and 2 children

THIS IS ONE OF MY ALL-TIME FAVORITE SOUPS. DEPENDING ON WHETHER you like your soup sweet or savory, you can flavor it with either orange juice or *brodo* (page 301). The baked garlic is so mellow that you barely notice it. The sage adds a nutty taste, and the fried sage leaf garnish is a fun twist.

This soup freezes well, but make the crispy sage garnish right before serving.

2 small butternut squash, halved lengthwise and seeded, pulp discarded

3 tablespoons olive oil

2 cloves garlic, halved (optional)

1 tablespoon salted butter

1 large onion, chopped

2 chopped fresh sage leaves plus 10 whole fresh sage leaves

1½ cups orange juice

1½ cups *Brodo* (page 301) or ready-to-use low-sodium vegetable broth

¼ teaspoon ground nutmeg

½ teaspoon dried thyme

1 teaspoon sea salt

½ teaspoon ground black pepper

1. Preheat the oven to 400°F.
2. Brush the bottom of a baking dish and the cut surfaces of the squash with the oil. Place half a clove of garlic, if using, inside each squash cavity and place the squash in the pan, cut-side down. Pour ½ cup of water into the pan, cover with foil, and bake in the oven for 40 to 50 minutes, or until the squash is tender when pricked with a fork.
3. Meanwhile, in a small skillet over medium heat, melt half of the butter. Add the

onions and chopped sage, and cook until the onions turn golden brown, 4 to 5 minutes. Transfer the onion mixture to a plate and set aside.

4. Make the crispy sage leaves: In the same skillet over medium heat, melt the remaining butter. Add the whole sage leaves and sauté until they are browned and slightly curled at the edges, about 3 minutes. Transfer the crispy sage leaves to a plate lined with paper towel (to absorb excess butter) and set aside.

5. Using a spoon, scoop out the flesh from the cooked squash and transfer it to a blender. Add the onion mixture, garlic, orange juice, *brodo*, nutmeg, thyme, salt, and pepper and purée until smooth. Ladle into bowls and garnish with one or two crispy sage leaves. (I sometimes sprinkle salt on the crispy sage leaves right before using them as a garnish to make them extra tasty.)

Ⓓ Mild Thai Squash Curry

45 minutes to prepare (10 minutes hands-on); serves 4 adults or 6 children

DON'T BE ALARMED BY THE WORD "CURRY"! I PROMISE THAT THIS IS A RECipe even cautious children will love. The sweet coconut offsets the mild taste of the ginger. It's a wonderful introduction to the world of curries.

2 cups Thai rice (or ½ cup per adult or older child)

3 large carrots, peeled and cut into bite-size pieces (about 2 cups)

1 small acorn squash, peeled, halved, seeded, and cut into bite-size pieces (about 3 cups)

1 large sweet potato, peeled and cut into bite-size pieces (about 2 cups)

1 tablespoon vegetable oil

1 clove garlic, halved

4 small boneless, skinless chicken breasts, cut into bite-size pieces

One 14-ounce can coconut milk

Juice of 1 lime (about 1 tablespoon)

½ teaspoon ground ginger

¼ teaspoon sea salt

1 teaspoon Thai curry paste

1 teaspoon liquid honey, packed dark brown sugar, or pure maple syrup

¼ cup finely chopped fresh cilantro leaves

1. Set a medium saucepan over medium heat with 4 cups of water (for the rice) and a large saucepan over high heat with 8 cups of water (for the vegetables).
2. When the water in the medium saucepan is boiling, add the rice, reduce the heat to low, cover, and cook for 20 minutes, or as directed on the package. (The rice is cooked when fluffy and the water is fully absorbed.)
3. Meanwhile, in the other saucepan, add the carrots, squash, and sweet potato, reduce the heat to medium-high, and simmer until the vegetables are just tender, about 5 minutes. Drain the vegetables.
4. In a large skillet over medium heat, heat the oil. Add the garlic and chicken and cook, stirring constantly, for 3 to 4 minutes, or until chicken is cooked through. Remove the garlic pieces. Add the cooked carrots, squash, and sweet potato, the coconut milk, lime juice, ginger, salt, and Thai curry paste. Cover and simmer for 12 to 15 minutes, or until the vegetables are tender. Stir in the honey and cilantro just before serving.

TOMATOES

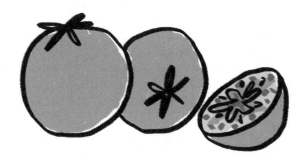

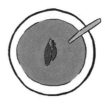

A TOMATO PEACH
BASIL PURÉE

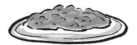

B ROCKSTAR RAGOUT

C PEEK-A-BOO
STUFFED TOMATOES
(TOMATES FARCIES)

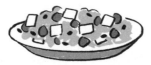

D TASTY TAGINE CASSEROLE

A # Tomato Peach Basil Purée (aka Baby Gazpacho)

8 minutes to prepare (2 minutes hands-on); makes 6 to 8 baby jars

THE FLAVORS OF TOMATO AND PEACH ARE A SURPRISINGLY WONDERFUL blend. The slightly sweet taste of the peach reduces the acidity of the tomatoes and lends a smooth creaminess to the purée. Bonus: this is the starting point for one of the world's best soups, Spanish gazpacho, a veggie-packed, super healthy, incredibly easy, no-cook cold summer soup. Think of it as the best veggie smoothie you ever tasted, and get ready to explore those tastes with your baby!

As with all of the other purée recipes, this makes a great adult soup, too. Double the recipe for each additional adult and garnish with a sprinkle of chopped basil.

This purée freezes well.

2 medium very ripe tomatoes, cored and chopped
1 or 2 fresh basil leaves, finely chopped
1 large or 2 small ripe peaches, pitted, peeled, and quartered

1. In a medium saucepan over medium-low heat, combine the tomatoes and basil with just enough water to cover the tomatoes. (The tomatoes will release more liquid while cooking.) Arrange the peaches on top of the tomatoes (so that they steam rather than boil—or they will get really mushy fast). Alternatively, steam the peaches in a separate saucepan using a steamer insert. Cook until the peaches are soft, about 5 minutes. Strain the tomatoes and peaches, reserving the cooking liquid.
2. Using a food processor or immersion blender, purée the tomatoes and peaches, adding enough cooking liquid to reach desired consistency.

Taste-Training Tip: As your baby grows, you can gradually convert this soup into a gazpacho. Introducing one new ingredient at a time as you accustom your baby to the tastes, add these ingredients before blending: 1 cup tomato juice, ½ cup chopped yellow or red bell pepper, ¼ cup finely chopped fresh parsley leaves, 2 tablespoons olive oil plus 1 tablespoon lemon juice (or ¼ cup orange juice), ¼ cup chopped onion, 1 tablespoon chopped fresh basil leaves, ¼ teaspoon sea salt, and ¼ teaspoon ground black pepper. Experiment with the flavor combinations you like best.

Ⓑ Rockstar Ragout

20 minutes to prepare (5 minutes hands-on); serves 2 adults (double the recipe for a family of 4)

RAGOUT (OR RAGÙ) IS ITALIAN COMFORT FOOD. THERE'S ALSO A FRENCH version of this dish (a slow-cooked stew, often served with potatoes), but I prefer the Italian approach by far. There are many variations on this stew, but I like my version plain and simple. The French name (*ragoût*) comes from the (ancient) word *ragoûter*, which translates as "to revive the taste" or "to stimulate the appetite." This dish certainly does that!

If you have an older child who doesn't enjoy eating meat, try them on this melt-in-your-mouth dish. Serve it with pasta sprinkled with Parmesan. *Delicious!*

This dish freezes well.

1 tablespoon olive oil

1 clove garlic, halved

½ pound high-quality ground beef

2 carrots, peeled and sliced into ½-inch coins

One 28-ounce can diced tomatoes or 2½ cups diced fresh tomatoes

3 tablespoons tomato paste

½ teaspoon chopped fresh flat-leaf parsley leaves

¼ teaspoon dried thyme

¼ teaspoon dried oregano

Sea salt and ground black pepper, optional

1. In a medium saucepan over medium-low heat, heat the oil. Add the garlic and sauté for 1 minute, or until brown. Add the ground beef, increase the heat to medium-high, and cook, stirring constantly, for 1 minute. Add the carrots and cook, stirring occasionally, for 3 to 4 minutes, or until the beef is cooked through. Stir in the tomatoes, tomato paste, parsley, thyme, and oregano. Cover, reduce the heat to medium, and simmer for 10 minutes, stirring occasionally.

2. Transfer the beef mixture to a food processor and purée (see Taste-Training Note). For adults or older children, you might want to season with salt and pepper.

Taste-Training Note: For younger babies who aren't yet chewing, you can purée the mixture until smooth. You can progressively transition them to more solid textures by setting aside part of the beef mixture before puréeing, and then stirring it into the purée before serving. Make it progressively chunkier as your baby grows, and they'll be eating "grown-up" ragout in no time!

 ## Peek-a-Boo Stuffed Tomatoes (*Tomates Farcies*)

55 minutes to prepare (15 minutes hands-on); serves 4 adults or older children (as a side dish)

I COULDN'T RESIST INCLUDING A READER'S FAVORITE RECIPE FROM *French Kids Eat Everything*. *Tomates farcies* are one of the most fun ways I know to serve tomatoes. They're stuffed with a savory ground beef mixture and then baked to perfection. The *farce* peeks out of the tomatoes in a coquettish sort of way; children love lifting up the tomato "hats" to see what lies underneath. Served with something that can absorb the delicious juices—rice and couscous are favorites—this is a nice, light, tasty meal.

2 tablespoons olive oil

1 small onion, minced

½ pound high-quality ground beef

4 large or 6 medium tomatoes

½ cup diced red or yellow bell pepper, optional

¼ cup dried breadcrumbs

½ teaspoon dried parsley or oregano, optional (see Notes)

¼ teaspoon sea salt

¼ teaspoon ground black pepper

¼ cup grated Parmesan cheese

1. Preheat the oven to 375°F.
2. In a medium skillet over low heat, heat the oil. Add the onion and sauté until golden brown, about 5 minutes. Increase the heat to medium-high, add the ground beef, and cook, stirring constantly, for 2 minutes or until lightly browned. Reduce the heat to medium-low and sauté until the beef is cooked through, 6 to 8 minutes.
3. Meanwhile, prepare the tomatoes: Slice off the tops and set them aside, then, using

a small spoon or melon baller, hollow out the insides of the tomatoes, transferring the pulp to a bowl. (The skins will look like little bowls.) Arrange the tomato "bowls" upside down on a plate and set aside to allow the juice to drain. Chop the reserved tomato pulp and add it to the simmering beef mixture along with the red pepper, if using.

4. In a small bowl, combine the breadcrumbs, parsley, and salt and pepper. Add the breadcrumb mixture to the beef mixture and stir well to combine.

5. Spoon the meat mixture (the "*farce*") into the tomato "bowls" and sprinkle with the Parmesan. Put the tops back on the tomatoes. Transfer the stuffed tomatoes to a baking dish and bake in the oven for 20 to 25 minutes, or until they are deliciously melt-in-your-mouth (*fondant*). Remove from the oven and cool for 5 minutes before serving.

Notes: This dish can easily be prepared the night before and refrigerated until ready to bake. If you put the tomatoes straight into the oven from the fridge, you'll need to increase the baking time to up to 30 minutes.

You can try this recipe using any herbs and spices you like—my sister-in-law uses paprika. Get creative!

Taste-Testing Tip: For younger babies still getting used to solid foods, you can combine about one third of a cooked tomato with some meat mixture, tomato paste, and a little water, and purée for a ready-to-eat ragout.

Ⓓ Tasty Tagine Casserole

25 minutes to prepare (5 minutes hands-on); serves 2 adults and 2 children

A TAGINE IS A NORTH AFRICAN VEGETABLE STEW—EATEN EVERYWHERE IN that region, in endlessly delicious variations (sort of like Asian stir-fries). Don't be put off by the fancy-sounding name; this is a simple dish that combines the savory flavor of meat (chicken) with sweet raisins and spices. It's another great dish to encourage reluctant meat-eaters, as the chicken is melt-in-your-mouth tender. *Yum!*

2 tablespoons olive oil
4 boneless, skinless chicken breasts, cut into bite-size pieces
1 small onion, diced

1 clove garlic, halved

¼ teaspoon ground ginger

¼ teaspoon ground allspice

½ teaspoon ground cinnamon

¼ teaspoon ground turmeric, optional

¼ teaspoon ground cumin, optional

4 carrots, peeled and cut into bite-size pieces (about 3 cups)

1 large zucchini, peeled and cut into bite-size pieces

2 large tomatoes, chopped

1 tablespoon tomato paste

½ cup orange juice

½ cup golden raisins

Sea salt and ground black pepper, optional

Cooked rice, polenta, couscous, or quinoa, for serving

Chopped fresh flat-leaf parsley leaves, optional

1. In a large saucepan or Dutch oven over medium heat, heat the oil. Increase the heat to high, add the chicken, and cook, stirring often, until lightly seared, about 3 to 4 minutes.

2. Reduce the heat to medium, add the onion, garlic, ginger, allspice, cinnamon, and turmeric and cumin, if using, and cook for 3 minutes, until the onion is just starting to turn golden brown. Add the carrots, zucchini, tomatoes, tomato paste, orange juice, and ½ cup of water. Increase the heat to high and bring the stew to a boil. Once boiling, cover, reduce the heat to low, and simmer for 10 minutes, stirring occasionally.

3. Add the raisins and salt and pepper, if using, and cook for 2 to 3 minutes, uncovered, until the sauce reduces slightly (it will still be quite watery). Serve with your desired grain or starch, sprinkled with parsley for a bit of color.

Taste-Training Tip: For smaller babies, purée a morsel or two of chicken with some carrots and a little of the sauce from the finished dish.

ZUCCHINI

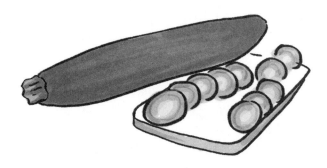

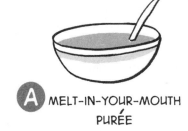

A MELT-IN-YOUR-MOUTH PURÉE

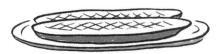

B ROASTED ZUCCHINI WITH CUMIN

C ZUCCHINI FLAN

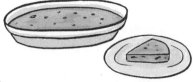

D QUICK ZUCCHINI-HAM QUICHE

Melt-in-Your-Mouth Zucchini Purée

7 minutes to prepare (5 minutes hands-on); makes 4 to 6 baby jars (depending on the size of your zucchini)

THIS IS ONE OF THE SIMPLEST PURÉES OF ALL TO MAKE FOR YOUR BABY (AND is often used as a starter purée in France). It literally melts in your mouth, and the texture is indescribably light and airy. For younger babies, you can serve this plain. For older babies (9 months and up), start experimenting by adding a little bit of cumin or allspice—just a pinch at first!

> 2 medium zucchini, peeled and cut into 2-inch chunks
> Pinch ground allspice or ground cumin, optional
> 1 teaspoon salted butter

1. Bring a medium saucepan half-filled with water to a boil over high heat. Add the zucchini, reduce the heat to medium-low, and simmer for 5 minutes, or until the zucchini is tender. Strain the zucchini, reserving the cooking liquid.
2. Using a food processor or blender, purée the zucchini with the allspice, if using, until smooth, adding enough cooking liquid to reach desired consistency (about ½ cup). Serve dabbed with butter.

I made the zucchini purée today and my 8-month-old devoured it! Her first taste of the big Z!

—BRANDY

 # Roasted Zucchini with Cumin

15 minutes to prepare (5 minutes hands-on); serves 2 adults and 2 kids (as a side dish)

WHEN YOUR CHILD IS READY TO CHEW SOLID FOODS, THIS IS A FUN WAY TO introduce them to roasted vegetables. The zucchini will become soft and tender in the oven, and the flavors of cumin and olive oil marry beautifully. (You can also cook these on the grill, but the oven version is tender and easier for children to chew.)

This also makes a nice adult side dish; just pop a few extra zucchini in the oven! Don't bother peeling the zucchini if you're serving it to older kids and adults.

1 large zucchini

1 clove garlic, halved, optional

1 teaspoon ground cumin

1 teaspoon sea salt, optional

2 tablespoons olive oil

1. Preheat the oven to 400°F.
2. Using a paring knife, peel the zucchini and remove the ends (no need to peel for adults), then cut it in half lengthwise. Make shallow criss-cross incisions across the cut sides of the zucchini and lay them, cut-side up, in a baking dish.
3. If using garlic, rub the halved clove over the cut side of the zucchini. Sprinkle with cumin and salt, if using (careful, you will need very little salt in this dish). Drizzle with oil. Add ½ cup of water to the baking dish. Bake in the oven for 5 minutes, flip zucchini over, and bake for 5 minutes more, or to desired tenderness.

I made the roasted zucchini tonight. I could not believe how tasty it was. So simple and so good! My 2½-year-old ate it without much encouragement. I will definitely make it again. It was great. I may even try it with the skin on next time. —BABETTE

Zucchini Flan

1 hour 10 minutes to prepare (15 minutes hands-on); serves 6 to 8 adults or children

THE FRENCH EAT FLANS OF ALL SORTS, BOTH SWEET AND SAVORY. FLANS are a great way to introduce children to the taste of baked eggs so they can move on to enjoying quiche with the whole family.

This simple recipe highlights the mild taste of the zucchini and combines it with onions that have been cooked until mild, rich, and melt-in-your-mouth. The touch of cumin adds a nice flavor without being overwhelming.

2 tablespoons olive oil

2 tablespoons salted butter

1 medium onion, very finely sliced

½ teaspoon ground nutmeg

5 or 6 fresh basil leaves, very finely chopped

Sea salt and ground black pepper, optional

4 medium zucchini, peeled and cut into 1/8-inch coins

1 teaspoon ground cumin

3 large eggs

⅔ cup whipping (35%) cream or ricotta cheese

½ cup shredded Cheddar cheese

½ cup grated Parmesan cheese

1. Preheat the oven to 400°F. Grease a baking dish with 1 tablespoon butter.

2. In a medium saucepan over medium heat, heat 1 tablespoon oil. Add 1 tablespoon butter, the onions, nutmeg, basil, and a pinch of salt, if using, and stir to combine. Cover and cook for 6 to 7 minutes, stirring occasionally, until the onions are tender.

3. Meanwhile, in a large skillet over medium-high heat, heat the remaining 1 tablespoon oil. Add the zucchini, sprinkle it with cumin, and cook for 5 minutes, stirring often, until just tender (do not overcook). Remove from the heat, drain any excess water, and sprinkle with salt and pepper, if using.

4. In a medium bowl, whisk together the eggs and cream. Set aside.

5. In the prepared baking dish, spread half the cooked onions in an even layer. Top with half the cooked zucchini, then half the cheese. Repeat the three layers with the remaining ingredients. Pour the egg mixture overtop, ensuring everything is evenly covered. (Cheese lovers might want to sprinkle a little extra Parmesan on top.)

6. Bake in the oven for 30 minutes, or until the vegetables are cooked through and the cheese is melted and browned. Remove from the oven and set aside to cool for 5 to 10 minutes. (This dish stays very hot in the center, and resting the flan will help the pieces slide out more easily.) To serve, cut the flan into slices.

~~~~~~~~~~~~~~~~~~~~~~~~~~~

Ⓓ Quick Zucchini-Ham Quiche

47 minutes to prepare (7 minutes hands-on); serves 2 adults and 2 children (with seconds)

EASY AND QUICK TO MAKE, THIS NO-CRUST VERSION OF CLASSIC FRENCH quiche will please adults and children alike. Quiche is versatile, as it can be eaten hot or cold, for lunch or for dinner, and with any combination of vegetables that you can think of.

This is a children's version of the recipe—it uses more milk and fewer eggs than a quiche intended for adults. The resulting dish is fluffier, less dense, and less eggy, and so more likely to please young palates. For older children and adults, reduce the milk by ½ cup and add 1 more egg (or play with the ratio of eggs and milk until you find the texture your family prefers).

10 large eggs
½ cup milk
½ teaspoon ground nutmeg
1 teaspoon ground cumin
Sea salt and ground black pepper, optional
1 cup grated Gruyère (preferred) or Cheddar cheese
1 cup cubed cooked ham or ½ cup crumbled cooked bacon
2 cups peeled and grated zucchini

1. Preheat the oven to 375°F. Grease a pie plate.
2. In a large bowl, beat the eggs lightly, then add the milk, nutmeg, and cumin and mix well. Add a pinch each of salt and pepper, if using. Stir in the cheese, then the ham and zucchini.
3. Pour the mixture into the prepared pie plate and bake in the oven for 30 to 40 minutes, or until a knife slid into the center comes out clean. Remove from the oven and set aside for 5 minutes to cool before serving (the quiche will settle, and you'll be able to cut it more neatly).

Taste-Training Tip: Changing your quiche ingredients is a great way to introduce new vegetables. The reassuringly familiar look of the dish will likely entice even the wariest of eaters to try a new, yummy vegetable. Once your child likes this version, try quiche with red peppers or even broccoli.

The flavor is quite subtle, but for a quick weeknight meal you can't go wrong with that. I served it to my husband and 2-year-old, and then proceeded to have a 15-minute uninterrupted conversation with my husband while my daughter quietly ate hers. She was hungry and it hit the spot! Love that! All in all, a hit.
—TERESA

APPLES

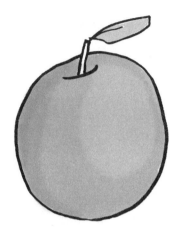

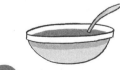
A SPICE IS NICE PURÉE

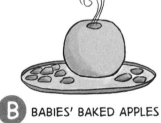
B BABIES' BAKED APPLES

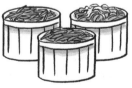
C SARAH'S SLAW SALAD

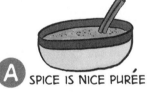
D CURRIED APPLE SOUP

Fun with Flavours!
Fruit Recipes

 Spice Is Nice Purée

10 minutes to prepare (5 minutes hands-on); makes 6 to 8 baby jars

MOST BABIES LOVE APPLES IN ANY FORM, SO THEY'RE A GREAT MEDIUM FOR introducing other flavors. In this purée, a little hint of ginger is combined with the teensiest bit of cinnamon. If desired, you can start with just cinnamon, or just ginger, instead of using both spices as called for in the recipe. Baby will get used to more variety and hopefully be more interested in the curry dishes you'll serve when they're older!

This purée freezes well.

4 apples, peeled, cored, and quartered (see Note)
¼ teaspoon ground cinnamon
Tiny pinch dried ginger
½ teaspoon fresh lemon juice, optional
Plain yogurt, for serving, optional

1. In a medium saucepan over medium-low heat, bring 1 cup of water to a boil. Add the apples, cover, and simmer until soft, 4 to 5 minutes. Strain the apples, reserving the cooking liquid. Transfer the cooked apples to a blender or food processor,

add the cinnamon and ginger, and purée. If you prefer a thinner purée, slowly add enough cooking liquid to reach desired consistency. If you prefer a tangier taste, add the lemon juice. Be sure to let the purée cool before serving—it will be hot! The purée is lovely with a little dollop of yogurt for a nice texture contrast.

Note: In this recipe, I prefer to use sweeter apples such as Fuji, Gala, Honeycrisp, or Pink Lady. Granny Smith or other sour apples don't work as well.

 ## Babies' Baked Apples

40 minutes to prepare (10 minutes hands-on); 1 apple per person

THIS DISH IS A READER FAVORITE FROM *FRENCH KIDS EAT EVERYTHING*. It's one of our favorite wintertime desserts and a real time-saver. I pop the apples in the oven before I start making dinner, and by the time the meal is ready to serve, the smell of the apples fills the house, luring the children to the table (at least, that's the theory!).

This recipe can be used to help transition babies to more solid foods. Baked long enough, the apple will have a texture as creamy as applesauce. Reduce the baking time, and the consistency gets progressively more solid.

1 apple per person, washed, stemmed, and cored, skin pricked with a fork
1 teaspoon pure maple syrup per apple, plus more for drizzling, optional (see Note)
Ground cinnamon, optional
Granulated sugar for sprinkling, optional

1. Preheat the oven to 375°F.
2. Arrange the apples upright in a baking dish and add ½ cup of water to the dish. Drizzle maple syrup into the hole in each apple (a little may seep out of the bottom). Dust with cinnamon, if using.
3. Bake the apples in the oven for about 25 to 30 minutes, or until they reach desired consistency. Just before serving, baste the apples with the sauce in the bottom of the dish. Serve the apples on individual plates, with maple syrup drizzled around the top of the apples or sprinkled with a bit of sugar and cinnamon.

Safety Tip: Be sure to let the apples cool down for at least 5 minutes before eating them. Just out of the oven, they will be piping hot inside and can burn little tongues. Don't judge whether the apple is cool enough to eat by how warm the peel is to the touch; the flesh inside will remain much hotter than the outside surface, which will cool down quite quickly. We cut the apples for our children and let the pieces cool on plates on the counter before bringing them to the table.

Note: To make this as the French do, substitute 1 tablespoon sugar and 1 tablespoon melted butter for the maple syrup. If using the butter/sugar combination, spoon it into the apple cores after they've been baking for about 15 minutes.

My daughter would like me to tell you it was the "best baked apple she has ever eaten." She's never had one before, and she wasn't enthusiastic about the concept, but she loved every last bite. Even my other daughter, my non-food adopter, ate her entire apple. I could see this as a staple recipe at our house. —LORI

I made the baked apples last night for the toddlers and the rest of my family, and they were a huge hit with everyone! The apples were delicious on their own, but we made it a party and added a scoop of vanilla ice cream. I have a feeling I'll be making this all winter long. —MEG

 ## Sarah's Slaw Salad

10 minutes to prepare (10 minutes hands-on); serves 2 adults and 2 to 4 children (as a side salad)

I CREATED THIS RECIPE FOR SARAH, ONE OF THE MORE RELUCTANT KIDS WHO TASTE tested the recipes in this book with me. It's a great way to introduce children to coleslaw: it uses apples, carrots, and only a small amount of cabbage (at first). The oil and vinegar dressing is a lighter alternative to the rich, creamy dressings often used in coleslaws. This salad also subtly introduces a new spice (cumin) that's one of the key ingredients in curry—preparing kids' taste buds for the curried soup that follows in this series.

2 apples, peeled, cored, and cut into bite-size pieces (I prefer Granny Smith)
2 large carrots, peeled and finely grated

1 tablespoon fresh lemon juice

½ cup raisins or currants, soaked in 1 cup warm water, optional

1 cup finely sliced purple (red) cabbage

Dressing:

3 tablespoons extra virgin olive oil

1 tablespoon balsamic vinegar or apple cider vinegar

½ teaspoon sea salt

¼ teaspoon ground cumin, optional

⅛ teaspoon ground cinnamon, optional

Optional Toppings:

1 shallot, minced

1 tablespoon roasted sunflower seeds

1 tablespoon minced fresh mint or parsley leaves or 1 teaspoon dried mint or parsley

1. In a bowl, combine the apples with the lemon juice to prevent browning.
2. If using the raisins, drain using a fine-mesh sieve, discarding the soaking water, and transfer to a large bowl. Add the cabbage, carrots, and prepared apples and mix to combine.
3. Make the dressing: In a small bowl, whisk together the oil, vinegar, salt, and cumin and cinnamon, if using. (Note: the quantity of dressing is deliberately small, so that the salad is not overdressed. If you know you like this dressing, you can double the quantities.)
4. Add the dressing to the salad and toss to coat well. Sprinkle with your toppings of choice. Serve at room temperature or slightly chilled.

Taste-Training Tips: For kids who are still learning to like some of these foods, try this: announce a "buffet salad" starter for your meal and place small bowls of each sliced ingredient on the counter or table. Kids can serve themselves from each bowl and "mix" their own salad. The only rules are that (a) they have to take something from each bowl, and (b) they have to taste everything they've taken. This will give kids who balk at certain fruits or vegetables the sense of control they might be seeking, while still encouraging them to taste new things.

Start with the small amount of cabbage as per the recipe, but as the kids begin (hopefully) to like it, increase the amount of red cabbage gradually, until it is equal to the carrot.

My very picky 3-year-old son ate his entire portion and did not complain one bit! He didn't seem to mind the new taste of the cabbage. The entire thing was so easy and quick to put together—it took 10 minutes from start to finish. Will be going in our repertoire!—JESSICA

 ## Curried Apple Soup

30 minutes to prepare (10 minutes hands-on); serves 2 adults and 2 children

BEFORE I HAD CHILDREN, CURRIED APPLE-SQUASH SOUP WAS ONE OF MY favorites. So when I started introducing curry spices to my children, this seemed like the natural go-to dish. I've simplified it for busy parents but preserved the essence: sweet apples offset the savory soup with a hint of mild curry. After trial and error, I found that this works best with juicy, tart apples (such as Spartan, McIntosh, or Granny Smith). The flavors in this soup will intensify if made a few hours prior to the meal (or even the night before).

This is a great lunch soup; just pack it in thermoses and go! I also make large batches and freeze them in quantities appropriate for one family meal. Then I simply remove what I need from the freezer in the morning; by dinnertime, the soup is thawed and ready to be gently heated and enjoyed.

1 tablespoon butter

1 tablespoon olive oil

½ cup chopped onion or leek, white part only

1 large yam, peeled and chopped

1 cup chopped celery or celeriac

2 cups peeled, cored, chopped apples

1 to 2 teaspoons curry powder, to taste

½ teaspoon ground ginger or 1 teaspoon freshly grated gingerroot

4 cups *Brodo* (page 301) or ready-to-use low-sodium vegetable or chicken broth

2 bay leaves

1 teaspoon sea salt, optional

1 cup half-and-half (10%) cream (for a rich soup) or whole milk (for a lighter soup)

1. In a large saucepan over medium-low heat, melt the butter in the olive oil. Add the onion and celery and sauté for 5 minutes. Add the apples, yam, curry powder, and ginger, reduce the heat to medium, and sauté for 3 minutes, until the apples are just tender. Add the *brodo,* bay leaves, and salt, if using. Increase the heat to high and bring to a boil. Once boiling, reduce the heat to medium and simmer until the celery is tender, 6 to 8 minutes. Remove from the heat. Discard the bay leaves.

2. Using a food processor or blender, purée the soup. Return the soup to the pot, if necessary, then stir in the cream. Taste and add more salt, if desired. Reheat the soup if necessary—but *gently* (don't let it boil).

Serving Tip: After pouring the soup into bowls, swirl in a small spoonful of light cream, sour cream, or plain yogurt, or sprinkle with a small pinch of dried thyme or mint for a decorative effect.

The flavor of this soup is out of this world—it could be served in a five-star restaurant. I was worried that my husband would freak out about this recipe, as he never likes fruit in his savory food. Well . . . he loved it. —BABETTE

My 7-year-old is my pickiest eater. He dipped some bread in the soup to taste it and gave it a "B+"! —STACY

I'm completely new to cooking, but the soup is quite straightforward to do, and so smooth to eat, yet new and interesting with a variety of flavors. My kids gobbled it down so fast without complaining once, I was blown away! —FRANÇOISE

AVOCADOS

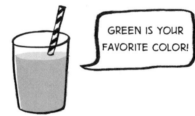

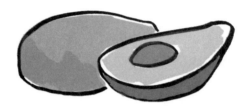

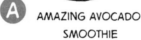

A AMAZING AVOCADO SMOOTHIE

B BEGINNER'S GUACAMOLE

C AWESOME AVOCADO ICE POPS

D AVOCADO SALSA SALAD

Amazing Avocado Smoothie

5 minutes to prepare (5 minutes hands-on); serves 2 adults and 2 children

Rich, satisfying, and super-nutritious, avocados are a quick and easy go-to option for parents. Although we tend to think of avocados as ingredients in savory dishes (such as guacamole), they're often served sweetened in other parts of the world (avocado ice cream!). Avocado's versatility makes it a great base from which to introduce your child to lots of different flavors and textures.

This smoothie is easy to make in the mornings and has now become a family breakfast favorite on school days. My kids love peeling the bananas and taking turns deciding what fruit to add. For cautious or reactive eaters, this can actually be a useful strategy: they'll be more willing to try "their" creation. You can enjoy this thick (eat it with a spoon) or thin (sip it through a straw), as desired, by varying the amounts of liquids you add.

> 1 cup fruit juice
> ½ cup water
> 1 avocado, peeled and pitted (see Note)
> 1 ripe banana
> Juice of ½ lemon (about 1 tablespoon)
> ½ cup cubed fresh or frozen peaches, optional

1. In a blender or food processor, combine the juice, water, avocado, banana, lemon juice, and peaches, if using, and purée until smooth.

Note: Avocado can sometimes have a slightly bitter aftertaste if really ripe, so I don't use overly ripe avocados. If you do, you might want to add 1 teaspoon of maple syrup or another ½ banana. Don't skip the lemon juice: avocado needs something acidic to balance the flavors.

Taste-Training Tip: Be inventive with this recipe. Instead of milk, try 1½ cups orange juice (skip the lemon juice) plus ½ cup plain yogurt. Part of the fun for kids is seeing how different ingredients result in different textures and tastes, so let them experiment, too. My kids have managed to make only one or two undrinkable smoothies, and their experiments were always interesting. Note, though, that berries don't work very well in this recipe—at least not according to our daughters and the test families!

Peeling avocados is easy

Using a sharp knife, cut the avocado lengthwise through the skin, all the way to the pit, all the way around. You now have two halves, still stuck together. Hold each half and twist in opposite directions. It should separate easily, and you will be able to lift one half off. The pit will remain in the other half. Whack the pit carefully with the sharp edge of the knife (so that it "bites" into the pit) and then lift the pit out. While the skin is still on, slice (or dice) the avocado flesh, then scoop it out with a spoon. (You can also find some good videos online that explain this technique.)

Even though it was her first food and a favorite from the beginning, my toddler daughter is in a state of total avocado refusal right now. But I was able to get her to try the smoothie, which she loved.

—BRANDY

The smoothie was the most beautiful shade of green I've ever seen! Our 10-year-old gave it a "10" on a scale of 1 to 10 (but then added he'd give it a "12" if he could go up higher).

—STACY

 Beginner's Guacamole

5 minutes to prepare (5 minutes hands-on); makes 2 baby jars

GUACAMOLE IS A GREAT DISH FOR KIDS—PACKED FULL OF HEALTHY VEGgies—and it's probably one of the easiest recipes in this book. Start off by serving plain avocado to your baby (directly out of the avocado half using a spoon is the easiest way). You can then start adding the ingredients below, one by one, until baby is eating something that fairly closely resembles adult guacamole. See the stages listed below for three versions for children of increasing ages.

We usually double this recipe to make a small side dish for our family.

1 ripe avocado

1 tablespoon sour cream or yogurt

¼ teaspoon orange or lime juice

¼ cup finely diced tomato

⅛ cup finely diced fresh cilantro leaves

¼ teaspoon ground cumin

1 tablespoon finely minced red or yellow onion

Stage 1: Serve the avocado plain or, for older babies (1 year or older), serve half an avocado on a plate, with the little "bowl" (made by removing the pit) filled with a dip or dressing that they like. I use the Classic Vinaigrette (page 302); the mild acidity perfectly offsets the rich, creamy avocado taste.

Stage 2: Peel and pit the avocado. In a food processor, combine the avocado with the sour cream and orange juice and purée.

Stage 3: Follow the instructions for Stage 2 above, then stir in the tomato. Once your child likes this version, add the cilantro. Once that has been accepted, add the cumin. Finish with the minced onion. *Voilà*: guacamole!

Taste-Training Tip: If you have children at different stages, you can also place these ingredients in separate bowls on the table and invite the kids to mix their own guacamole. Adventurous eaters will use more ingredients, and kids who are still learning to like this dish will experience some low-pressure positive peer encouragement as they see the others trying and enjoying the various ingredients.

The guacamole recipe is terrific. I usually just mash it up with lime, salt, and cumin, but the additional items were so delicious that I will definitely add them to my list.   —BRANDY

I really loved the idea of using the avocado as a bowl, so I just chopped up tomatoes and cilantro and served it with a vinaigrette. At first my 3-year-old said it was "yucky," but then he tried it—the big hurdle being getting him to put the salsa and avocado on the spoon and eat it all at the same time. It got a "yummy"!   —MARTHA

Awesome Avocado Ice Pops

2 hours 5 minutes to prepare (5 minutes hands-on); at least 6 big (double) ice pops

ICE POPS ARE AN AMAZING WAY TO INTRODUCE NEW FLAVORS TO YOUR KIDS. We enjoy them throughout the summer (and homemade ones are so much cheaper than store-bought). This recipe is adapted from Fany Gerson's *Paletas* cookbook, which features recipes for tropical ice pops and shaved ice inspired by the flavors of Mexico and including everything from tamarind and hibiscus flower to strawberry. If this recipe inspires you, those in her cookbook are a great next step.

> 1 large ripe avocado, halved, pitted, and peeled
> ⅓ cup grape or apple juice
> ⅓ cup coconut milk
> 2 tablespoons fresh lime juice
> Pinch sea salt
> ¼ cup berries, optional

1. In a food processor, combine the avocado, grape juice, coconut milk (do not use coconut cream), lime juice, salt, berries, if using, and ⅓ cup of water and purée. Pour into an ice-pop mold and freeze.

 Avocado Salsa Salad

10 minutes to prepare (10 minutes hands-on); serves 2 adults and 2 children (with plenty of leftovers)

THIS IS A TASTY AND SLIGHTLY UNUSUAL TEXTURE COMBINATION THAT IS also super-good for you: research has shown that adding avocado to salads and/or salsa can increase your intake of nutrients. This is because some nutrients are fat-soluble, and avocados have a relatively high proportion of (healthy) fats (in fact, they're one of the only fruits that do).

This is a great summer salad recipe, with contrasting colors and textures. On hot days, we sometimes eat this with bread as our main meal at lunchtime.

2 ripe but still firm avocados, halved, pitted, peeled, and cut into 1-inch cubes

2 tablespoons fresh lime juice

1 tablespoon minced fresh cilantro leaves, optional

¼ teaspoon sea salt

1 small head romaine or green leaf lettuce, torn into bite-size pieces

½ red or green bell pepper, cored, seeded, and diced

½ small red onion, finely diced

4 ripe plum tomatoes, chopped, or 12 cherry tomatoes, halved

¼ cup hulled raw sunflower seeds, optional

1 tablespoon extra virgin olive oil

1. In a small bowl, combine the avocado with 1 tablespoon of the lime juice and the cilantro, if using. Season with salt and set aside.
2. In a large bowl, combine the lettuce, red pepper, onion, tomatoes, and sunflower seeds, if using. Add the remaining 1 tablespoon lime juice and the olive oil and toss to combine. Just before serving, spoon the avocado mixture on top of the salad and *lightly* toss to combine (adding the avocado mixture at the end and handling it gently will keep the avocado from getting mushy).

Taste-Training Tip: For toddlers or older kids reluctant to eat salad, try making sure they get smaller pieces of lettuce on their plate. Some kids start with the "crunchy" parts of lettuce leaves (the central spine of the leaf), which seem to be easier to chew than the more floppy, textured ends of the leaves.

My 4½-year-old loved it, and my 2½-year-old loved all but the lettuce part (which is typical for her). We ended up having "Mexican food night" at our house thanks to this delicious salad.
                                                                                —Babette

BERRIES

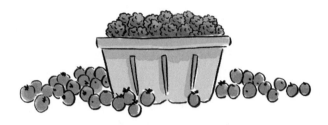

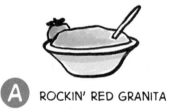

A ROCKIN' RED GRANITA

B BLACKBERRY SUPER SALAD

C PERFECT BLUEBERRY PARFAIT

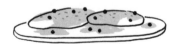

D SWEET AND SOUR
BLUEBERRY-GLAZED CHICKEN

Rockin' Red Granita

1 hour 15 minutes to prepare (10 minutes hands-on); serves 6 adults or children

RASPBERRIES ARE A WONDERFUL FRUIT FOR INTRODUCING TANGY FLAVORS to children. Their sweetness is naturally offset by just a hint of acidity—a little "zing" that adds a nice touch to this dish. The recipe also uses tomatoes, which balance out the sweetness of the raspberries (and they're much cheaper per pound, making this a reasonably priced berry dish; just make sure the tomatoes are ripe).

This recipe is served cold, which will be a new experience for many babies. It's perfect for a hot summer day. Think of this as a healthy equivalent to sorbet for little ones!

1 cup raspberries
½ pound ripe tomatoes, chopped
¼ cup peach or apple juice
2 teaspoons finely chopped fresh mint leaves
6 to 8 whole fresh mint leaves, for garnish

1. In a food processor, lightly process the raspberries, tomatoes, fruit juice, and chopped mint (see Note).
2. Transfer the berry mixture to a small saucepan, set over medium heat, and simmer for 5 minutes, stirring constantly. Divide the mixture evenly among 6 small bowls and set aside to cool (you can also freeze it in one large container, but it may take longer). Once cooled, freeze for about 45 minutes to 1 hour, stirring a few times, until just frozen. Using a fork or spoon, break up the granita. Garnish with mint leaves and serve. If you have extra raspberries, use them as a garnish.

Note: Smaller babies will need the granita to be very smooth; older babies may prefer it slightly chunky. For younger babies, you may want to strain the mixture through a fine-mesh sieve to remove the tomato seeds (I don't bother doing this).

I took a bite and thought, "This is different. Maybe I don't like this." But then I took a second bite, and I couldn't stop eating it. I finished my serving! —SARAH, AGE 8

Ⓑ Blackberry Super Salad

1 hour 10 minutes to prepare (10 minutes hands-on); serves 2 adults and 2 children

THIS IS A FUN TAKE ON A FRUIT SALAD THAT CAN BE SERVED AS A STARTER or dessert. The ginger gives it a little bit of bite that is offset by the sweetness of the fruit. It's a fun way to introduce your kids to "sharp" tastes. The thyme is an interesting contrast with the sweetness of the fruit and the spiciness of the ginger. This will be an unusual set of flavors for most children, so don't be surprised if they say "I don't like it" at first. It usually means "I don't know it yet." For more reluctant eaters, the honey syrup will help make things go a little more smoothly. Don't give up on the first try!

Honey Syrup (optional):
1 tablespoon liquid honey, pure maple syrup, or granulated sugar
½ cup water

Salad:
4 fresh, ripe peaches and/or nectarines, pitted, peeled, and chopped
½ cup blackberries or blueberries
1 teaspoon minced fresh thyme leaves
1 teaspoon lemon zest
2 tablespoons fresh lemon juice
½ teaspoon grated fresh gingerroot, optional

1. To make the Honey Syrup, if using: In a small saucepan over medium-high heat, combine the honey and water and bring it to a boil. Reduce the heat to medium-low and simmer until the liquid is reduced by half, about 10 minutes. Remove from the heat and set aside to cool.
2. In a large bowl, combine the peaches and blackberries. Add the honey syrup, if using, then add the thyme, lemon zest and juice, and ginger, if using. Stir gently to combine (don't overmix). Refrigerate for 1 hour before serving.

Taste-Training Tip: If you're introducing ginger to your child for the first time, set aside a portion of this salad without the ginger and serve that first. If your child likes it, then offer them the ginger option. Ask your child about the taste of ginger.

Fun with Ginger

Here is a great activity to do with your child. Buy a piece of fresh gingerroot and then have your child investigate its smell and taste. Your child will be intrigued by how mild it smells with its peel on, but how spicy it tastes when it's peeled and sliced. For more reluctant kids, try first giving them something else with ginger (ginger cookies, gingerbread, candied ginger, even ginger ale), and then ask them to taste the fresh ginger to see if they can detect a similar flavor. Research shows that children are more likely to accept new flavors if they're introduced to the sources first. This is about taste familiarization, not actually eating the ginger, so do this activity at a time and place not associated with a meal.

Perfect Blueberry Parfait

5 minutes to prepare (5 minutes hands-on); serves 2 adults and 2 children

THE LAYERING IN THIS DESSERT IS AN ADAPTATION OF A POPULAR FRENCH tactic for quick, easy, yet visually enticing aperitifs or desserts: *verrines*. *Verre* means "glass" in French, and a *verrine* means "little glass"—usually a thin glass that shows off the layers nicely. The French get really creative: for example, avocado might be layered with shrimp or crab mousse and topped with bits of candied citrus. The layers are much thinner than in the classic North American parfait and look more elegant (in my opinion).

In this easy *verrine* recipe, the combination of blueberries and walnuts may seem a little odd, but that's the point: the moist, sweet blueberries are a nice complement to the dry, earthy flavor of the nuts. Note that a full-fat yogurt, such as Greek yogurt, works best to hold the layers.

Kids love helping to put this dessert together. It's quick and easy to prepare, and looks festive and fun. Perfect!

    2 cups frozen or fresh blueberries
    2 cups plain, vanilla, or raspberry Greek yogurt
    1 cup raw or glazed walnuts, chopped
    4 teaspoons granola, optional

1. If using frozen blueberries, microwave them on high in a microwave-safe bowl for about 60 seconds, or just until the juices start flowing. If using fresh blueberries, place them in a small saucepan with a tiny bit of water and simmer over medium-high heat for 2 to 3 minutes until just tender; cool before using.

2. Spoon a thin layer (about 2 tablespoons) of yogurt into each small glass. Top with a thin layer of blueberries. Add alternating layers of yogurt and blueberries until you're near the top of the glass. Finish with a layer of walnuts and granola, if using (great for breakfast!), and garnish with a few blueberries.

We eat this for breakfast. Our usual school morning breakfast is either a fried or hard-boiled egg, a piece of toast with either honey or apple butter, and a yogurt parfait. It's actually very fast. The girls never tire of the presentation.   —*Lori*

 ## Sweet and Sour Blueberry-Glazed Chicken

40 minutes to prepare (10 minutes hands-on); serves 2 adults and 2 children

CHICKEN IS OFTEN A FAMILY FAVORITE, BUT IT'S EASY TO FALL INTO A BIT OF a routine (nuggets, anyone?). This is a fun way to expand your children's repertoire: the sauce is just sweet enough to please most palates and contrasts nicely with the chicken. Bonus: the cooked chicken is moist, which will allow some kids who are resistant to chicken to really enjoy this dish.

2 tablespoons butter
2 tablespoons olive oil
Sea salt and ground black pepper, to taste
4 boneless, skinless chicken breasts or 1½ pounds skinless chicken legs

Sweet and Sour Blueberry Glaze:
¼ cup sliced onion or shallots
1 cup fresh or frozen blueberries, plus extra for garnish
⅓ cup balsamic vinegar
¼ cup pure maple syrup or Honey Syrup (page 258)
1 tablespoon chopped fresh rosemary or 1½ teaspoons dried rosemary

½ teaspoon sea salt

¼ teaspoon ground black pepper

1 teaspoon fresh lemon juice, optional

1 sprig fresh rosemary, for garnish

1. Preheat the oven to 375°F.

2. In a large skillet over medium-high heat, melt 1 tablespoon butter in 1 tablespoon oil. Season the chicken with salt and pepper. When the butter mixture is hot (sputtering), add the chicken and sear for 1 minute or until light golden brown, then flip and sear the other side. Transfer the chicken to a baking dish and set aside.

3. Make the blueberry glaze: To the same skillet over medium-high heat, melt the remaining 1 tablespoon butter in the remaining 1 tablespoon oil. Stir in the onions and cook until softened and translucent, 4 to 5 minutes. Add the blueberries, increase the heat to high, and cook for 2 minutes. Reduce the heat to medium and stir in the vinegar, maple syrup, and rosemary and season with ½ teaspoon salt and ¼ teaspoon pepper. Simmer for 10 minutes, or until the blueberries start to dissolve. (For a more tart sauce with a real "zing," add the lemon juice.)

4. Pour the blueberry mixture over the prepared chicken and bake in the oven for 15 to 20 minutes, or until the chicken is cooked through. Serve garnished with a sprig of fresh rosemary and dotted with blueberries, if desired.

This was a breakthrough: the first time our 8-year-old girl ate non-nugget, unbreaded chicken. As always, she liked the sweetness. My wife and I also really liked the flavor mix of the maple syrup, blueberries, and balsamic. —Jon

My husband and I loved it, and Sophia said "Yummm" (she picked off all the blueberries first, then ate the chicken). —Teresa

We get to have blueberries as our dinner! —Hayden, age 7

CANTALOUPE

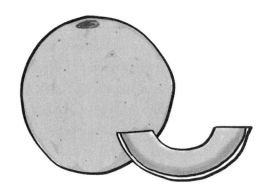

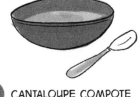 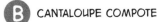

B CANTALOUPE COMPOTE

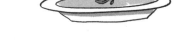 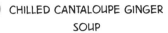

C CHILLED CANTALOUPE GINGER
SOUP

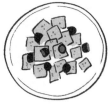

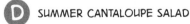

D SUMMER CANTALOUPE SALAD

Cantaloupe Compote

5 minutes to prepare (5 minutes hands-on); makes 6 to 8 baby jars

MELON IS OFTEN A KIDS' FAVORITE, AND MAKES FOR A WONDERFUL DESSERT. This compote is deliciously simple. When you serve cantaloupe to adults and older children (perhaps for a summer dessert), you can whip this up for baby.

This compote freezes well.

1 small ripe cantaloupe (see Note)

1. Using a sharp knife, cut the melon in half and, using a spoon, scoop out the seeds (discard seeds). Slice each half lengthwise to make "smile" (crescent) shapes. Cut the rind from each slice, then cut the slices into smaller chunks.
2. Transfer the cantaloupe to a blender and blend until smooth (it'll blend into a nice compote without the need for added liquid).

Note: A cantaloupe is ripe when its rind is pinkish-yellow rather than green and you can smell a fruity odor at the stem end.

Taste-Training Tip: Cantaloupe pairs wonderfully with raspberries and lemon or lime juice. As baby grows older, try experimenting with these flavor combinations.

Adult Serving Tip: Try this compote mixed with a little lemon or lime juice, served over ice cream, and topped with fresh basil leaves. Enjoy it with a glass of dessert wine.

Chilled Cantaloupe Ginger Soup

5 minutes to prepare (5 minutes hands-on); serves 6 adults or older children

ON THOSE SUMMER DAYS WHEN IT'S TOO HOT TO COOK, CHILLED SOUPS ARE a great choice: quick to make, hydrating, and refreshing. In fact, they're just a thin version of fruit smoothies, so you could always call this a smoothie. But the addition of basil and yogurt makes this creamy enough that I consider it a soup. You say *potayto*, I say *potahto*!

1 small ripe cantaloupe (see Note)

½ cup plain Greek yogurt

⅛ teaspoon ground ginger

Juice of 1 lime (about 2 tablespoons)

1 teaspoon liquid honey

2 or 3 fresh mint leaves or 1 tablespoon dried mint

2 or 3 fresh basil leaves or 1 tablespoon dried basil

Pinch sea salt

1. Using a sharp knife, cut the melon in half and, using a spoon, scoop out the seeds (discard seeds). Slice each half lengthwise to make "smile" (crescent) shapes. Cut the rind from each slice, then cut the slices into smaller chunks.

2. In a blender, combine the cantaloupe with the yogurt, ginger, lime juice, honey, mint, basil, and salt and purée until smooth. (You may need to add a few tablespoons of water to reach desired consistency.) Serve cold, in pretty little bowls. A little extra chopped basil or mint sprinkled on top will add the perfect touch.

Note: A cantaloupe is ripe when its rind is pinkish-yellow rather than green and you can smell a fruity odor at the stem end.

Summer Cantaloupe Salad

5 minutes to prepare (5 minutes hands-on); serves 4 adults or older children

Now that you've incorporated cantaloupe into your daily routine (or even if you haven't), try branching out! The acidity of the tomatoes and lime (and raspberries, if using) make this salad shine. Bonus: blend leftovers together and freeze to make a granita (see page 257).

Kids love to make this salad!

1 small ripe cantaloupe (see Notes)

1 cup cherry tomatoes, halved

¼ cup chopped fresh mint leaves

Juice of 1 lime or ½ lemon (about 1 tablespoon)

⅛ teaspoon ground ginger, optional (see Notes)

½ cup raspberries, for garnish, optional

1. Using a sharp knife, cut the melon in half and, using a spoon, scoop out the seeds (discard seeds). Slice each half lengthwise to make "smile" (crescent) shapes. Cut the rind from each slice, then cut the slices into smaller chunks.
2. In a large bowl, combine the cantaloupe, tomatoes, mint, lime juice, and ginger, if using, and toss lightly to combine. Garnish with raspberries, if desired.

Notes: A cantaloupe is ripe when its rind is pinkish-yellow rather than green and you can smell a fruity odor at the stem end.

If you use the ginger, whisk it into the lime juice first, before adding it to the salad.

CITRUS

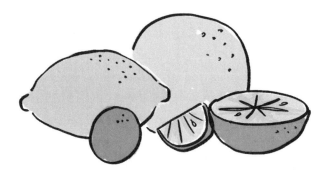

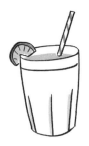

B TANGY CITRUS SMOOTHIE

WE LOVE SOUR!

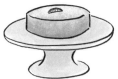

C ORANGE OLIVE OIL CAKE

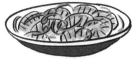

D ZESTY ORANGE SALAD

Tangy Citrus Smoothie

4 minutes to prepare (4 minutes hands-on); serves 2 adults and 2 children (small "tasting" servings)

SMOOTHIES (JUST LIKE SOUPS) ARE A GREAT WAY TO INTRODUCE NEW FLAVORS to your kids. The creamy, smooth texture makes them a natural hit with kids of all ages. Plus, they're versatile: my test families served this recipe for breakfast, snack, and dessert!

Note: I wouldn't recommend serving this before a child is 12 months old, and then only in small quantities (and test these ingredients, one by one, with your child first to watch for any allergic reactions). If they do react, best to wait. My older daughter used to react to tomatoes (a red rash around the mouth), and my younger one to kiwis. This eventually went away by itself. No rush! This recipe is very flexible, so you can mix and match ingredients. Kids love experimenting in the kitchen, and coming up with "their" smoothie recipe is a lot of fun (and a great way to get them taste testing).

By the way, if you don't like smoothies, this recipe might change your mind. My test families report that those who don't like the standard smoothie flavors (such as berry) were surprised to find the citrus to be so tasty.

1 cup orange juice
Juice of ½ lemon (about 1 tablespoon)
1 big or 2 small ripe bananas
½ cup plain yogurt (use flavored if your kids are not yet citrus lovers)
One of the following: half a peeled grapefruit, 1 peeled kiwi, or 1 cup diced pineapple
2 ice cubes
2 tablespoons liquid honey
1 ripe avocado, pitted and peeled, optional (see Taste-Training Tips)

1. In a blender, combine the orange juice, lemon juice, banana, yogurt, your choice of fruit, ice cubes, honey, and avocado, if using, and blend until smooth and frothy.

Taste-Training Tips: Smoothies concentrate flavors, making them more intense. For younger kids or those new to tangy tastes, this smoothie will probably need the flavored yogurt as well as the avocado, which will reduce the acidity level and balance the sour taste, making it interesting rather than overly strong.

I serve this recipe in mini, kid-size teacups or tall, thin juice glasses (or even cocktail glasses). This is a "tasting" recipe, so kids don't need a lot.

I chose the kiwi option because I love kiwi, but my three kids refuse to eat it. When I was preparing it, my pickiest eater said, "Mom, I warn you, I won't eat it if there's kiwi!" It was so easy to make, and I put it in tiny cocktail glasses so it would be fun. Both my 9- and 6-year-old hesitated, sipped a little, then gobbled it down. The 3-year-old didn't touch it, so her sister told her, "Tómalo, está riquísimo!" which means "Try some, it's really delicious!" We laughed! The eldest had three glasses, and even the youngest sipped twice and said, "Okay, it's good!" —FRANÇOISE

I made the smoothie tonight as our dessert. I used pineapple and poured it into tiny glasses with a bendy straw. The girls loved it so much! —LORI

 ## Orange Olive Oil Cake

40 minutes to prepare (10 minutes hands-on); makes 8 slices

MAKING A CAKE WITH OLIVE OIL IS NOT A NEW IDEA, BUT THAT DOESN'T make this recipe any less worth including. This is one of my favorite cake recipes of all time. Tangy yet sweet, this cake has the best flavor after it has sat for a day.

2 large eggs
⅔ cup granulated sugar
½ cup olive oil
1 tablespoon orange zest (see Taste-Training Tip)
Juice of 1 orange (about ½ cup)
¼ cup poppy seeds, optional
1½ cups all-purpose flour, plus more for dusting
1 tablespoon baking powder
¼ teaspoon sea salt
Confectioners' (icing) sugar, for sprinkling

1. Preheat the oven to 350°F. Grease and flour an 8-inch round cake pan.

2. In a large bowl, using an electric mixer on medium-high speed, mix the eggs and sugar until pale and fluffy, 3 to 4 minutes. With the mixer on, gradually add the olive oil in a thin stream, mixing until fluffy and light. Add the orange zest, orange juice, and poppy seeds, if using, and mix until well combined.

3. In a medium bowl, combine the flour, baking powder, and salt. With the mixer on low speed, add half the dry ingredients to the wet ingredients, mix until combined, then add the remaining dry ingredients and mix until just combined (don't overmix).

4. Pour the batter into the prepared cake pan and bake for 30 minutes, or until the top springs back when touched. Remove the pan from the oven, allow to cool slightly, then turn out onto a wire rack and set aside to cool completely. To serve, sprinkle with confectioners' sugar and cut into wedges. This cake stores beautifully for up to a week in the fridge or for a few days stored in an airtight container at room temperature.

Taste-Training Tip: For kids who are cautious about citrus, make this cake with the orange juice only, then gradually introduce the orange zest. The cake will be tangier (but not sour). This is a great way to introduce them to bitter tastes.

This was super easy to make! My 6-year-old daughter loved it. First she said, "Deeeeliciouuuus," then, "Buttery and salty and sweet, and I like the crust part the best." —ANALIS

We had the Orange Olive Oil Cake for snack this afternoon, and it was very good. I loved the tanginess of the orange. Sophia (2 years old) inhaled it: she votes with her mouth! —TERESA

Ⓓ Zesty Orange Salad

15 minutes to prepare (5 minutes hands-on); serves 2 adults and 2 children

THIS IS ONE OF THE RECIPES IN *FRENCH KIDS EAT EVERYTHING*, AND I couldn't resist introducing it again here. It's a dessert salad, which is a great way to introduce new flavors to children. The sweetness of the orange offsets the bitterness of the orange zest. Children will be reassured by the familiar (the pieces of orange) and so hopefully will be more willing to try something new (the thin, almost playful curlicues of sweetened orange rind).

Have your children watch you prepare this dish and let them try a sample if they're curious. When serving, remember that eating can sometimes be about encountering new tastes rather than consuming large quantities.

Serve this dish in a quiet moment when you have the time to sit and discuss the ingredients with your child. Questions are usually helpful (and helpfully distracting): How does the orange zest taste? Does it taste orangey at all? How does it taste when you nibble a tiny bit? Place a tiny piece on your tongue? What does it smell like? If your child doesn't want to eat any, that's fine, too, but encourage them to taste it.

Our daughters graduated from eating this salad to eating grapefruit, which they now enjoy as a breakfast treat. Claire, our younger daughter, will purse her lips and say, "Ooohhh, *Maman, c'est amer!* (it's bitter!)," and then continue eating with delight.

Because of its sweetness, the French would serve this as a dessert, even though it's called a salad.

4 seedless oranges
4 tablespoons granulated sugar

1. Wash 1 orange, dry it, and use a zester to peel all of the zest. (If you don't have a zester, use a sharp paring knife to carefully peel the outer layer, taking only the very outside of the rind and avoiding the white pith underneath. Slice the zest into very thin strips. Extra points for making curlicues by slicing around the orange.)
2. In a small saucepan over low heat, combine ½ cup of water and the sugar and cook for 5 minutes, stirring often, until the sugar is completely dissolved. Add the zest and simmer for 10 minutes, or until the zest is tender (the syrup may start to turn a golden color, which is fine).
3. Meanwhile, peel the remaining oranges, completely cutting off and discarding any pith so that you are left with just the fruit itself. Slice the oranges crosswise into thin circles and divide them evenly among 4 small salad bowls. Pour the zest and syrup overtop. Serve immediately.

In sum: possibly one of the best things I've ever tasted myself, and my kids licked their plates clean and asked for more. 'Nuff said!
—MARTHA

PEACHES

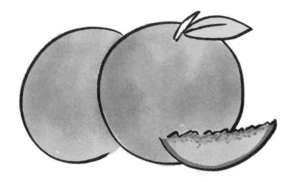

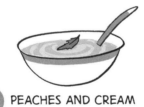

A PEACHES AND CREAM PURÉE

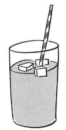

B LOVELY PEACHY MINT LEMONADE

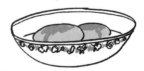

C "MAGIC SPICE" POACHED PEACHES

D SAVORY PEACH SALAD

Peaches and Cream Purée

4 minutes to prepare (2 minutes hands-on); makes 3 to 4 baby jars

BABY FRUIT PURÉES TEND TO GET A LITTLE REPETITIVE. USING PEACHES AS your base is a great way to introduce little palates to the taste of a slightly more acidic fruit. Peaches and cream is a wonderful taste combination for adults, and this recipe follows the same flavor principle for baby.

> 1 ripe peach, peeled and quartered
> 1 teaspoon half-and-half (10%) cream or whipping (35%) cream, or 1 tablespoon plain
>   Greek yogurt
> ⅛ teaspoon ground cinnamon

1. In a saucepan over high heat, bring 2 cups of water to a boil. Once boiling, add the peaches and cook for about 2 minutes, or until tender. Remove the pan from the heat and strain the peaches, reserving the cooking liquid. (It will already smell wonderful by now.)
2. In a blender, combine the cooked peaches, cream, and cinnamon and purée until smooth, adding enough cooking liquid to reach desired consistency. Enjoy!

Taste-Training Tip: For older babies, try varying the flavor. In place of the cinnamon, add ⅛ teaspoon ground ginger, 1 teaspoon lemon or orange juice, ¼ teaspoon dried mint, or just the tiniest bit of pure vanilla extract.

Adult Serving Tip: This purée makes a great sauce to serve with vanilla ice cream. Make 1 batch of the recipe for every two people and blend away! Garnish with fresh mint leaves—mint and peach are a nice flavor combination.

 ## Lovely Peachy Mint Lemonade

15 minutes to prepare (5 minutes hands-on); makes 2 to 3 cups

EVEN HUMBLE LEMONADE CAN ACT AS A VEHICLE FOR NEW AND FUN TASTES. Who would have thought this taste combination would work? But it does, to perfection.

(Confession: I sometimes make this using store-bought lemonade. If you don't feel like squeezing all of those lemons, it's an option.)

    2 peaches, peeled, pitted, and chopped
    ¼ cup granulated sugar
    ½ cup chopped fresh mint leaves
    Juice of 8 lemons (about 1 cup)
    ½ lemon, thinly sliced, for garnish
    ¼ cup whole mint leaves, for garnish

1. In a small saucepan over high heat, combine the peaches, sugar, chopped mint leaves, and 1 cup of water and bring to a boil, stirring constantly. When the sugar has dissolved, after about 2 minutes, reduce the heat to medium-low and simmer for 5 more minutes. Remove the pan from the heat and set aside to cool, then transfer the syrup to an airtight container and refrigerate (see Note).

2. Using a fine-mesh sieve set over a pitcher half-filled with ice cubes, strain the syrup (discard the solids). Add 2 cups of water (or more as desired) and the lemon juice. Serve garnished with the lemon slices and whole mint leaves.

Note: This simple peach-mint syrup is best when made in advance and chilled. It will keep for up to 2 weeks in the fridge.

Adventurous Eating Tip: Try substituting basil for the mint—trust me, it's tasty!

"Magic Spice" Poached Peaches

25 minutes to prepare (5 minutes hands-on); serves 4 adults or older children

POACHED FRUIT IS ONE OF OUR FAMILY'S FAVORITE DESSERTS. SURE, THERE are more elegant ways to serve peaches, but this is a fast dessert to make, can be served hot or cold, and, when properly garnished, looks rather elegant, too. My younger daughter, Claire, calls this the "magic spice" recipe because of the star anise. And she's right: star anise does look a little magical (at least to a 5-year-old in "fairy mode"). The bonus: you can use frozen peaches. We buy fresh peaches when they're sold by the case at the end of the summer, halve them, remove the pits, peel them, and freeze them in freezer bags. This way, we can poach them directly from the freezer. You can also buy frozen peaches at the grocery store.

½ cup packed dark brown sugar (see Notes)

One 2- to 3-inch cinnamon stick or 1 teaspoon ground cinnamon

3 whole star anise

¼-inch piece fresh gingerroot, peeled and thinly sliced or 1 teaspoon ground ginger

4 ripe peaches, quartered (see Notes)

½ cup slivered almonds, optional

1. In a medium saucepan, combine the brown sugar, cinnamon, star anise, and ginger with 3 cups of water. Bring to a boil over high heat, stirring often. Reduce the heat to medium-low and simmer, stirring occasionally, for about 10 minutes (the mixture will darken, and the flavors will slowly infuse the liquid). Add the peaches in a single layer. Cover and simmer for 5 minutes. Using a spoon, gently turn the peaches over, cover, and simmer for another 5 minutes, or until tender. Remove the pan from the heat, leaving the peaches in the syrup and the lid firmly on to prevent the syrup from getting too thick, and set aside for 10 minutes. (The heat will gradually cook the peaches, but they'll stay firm.)

2. Meanwhile, in a small, dry skillet over medium-high heat, toast the almond slivers, if using, until golden, 3 to 4 minutes (stir them often to avoid burning).

3. There are many ways to serve this dish. Try drizzling the cooked peaches with cream or spooning them over ice cream. Garnish with the toasted almonds. (If you add raspberry syrup and serve the peaches with ice cream, you'll be recreating the famous French dessert peach Melba, which renowned chef Auguste Escoffier created in honor of the Australian soprano singer Nellie Melba. *Ooh la la!*)

Notes: I like to use fine cane sugar in this recipe, but sugar substitutes such as stevia also work well.

Gourmet cooks will remove the peach skins using exotic methods like plunging them in boiling water. If you have the time and energy, go for it! Personally, out of sheer laziness, I often poach the peaches with the skins still on. They hold together nicely, and the kids don't seem to mind.

Ⓓ Savory Peach Salad

5 minutes to prepare (5 minutes hands-on); serves 4 adults or older children

I KNOW, I KNOW. YOU'RE PROBABLY THINKING, *ARUGULA, FOR MY KIDS? Are you kidding?* Well, trust me and try this recipe. Italian kids grow up eating the stuff. If you introduce arugula early enough, they'll take to it like ducks to water. To get started, take a gradual approach. If your kids are enjoying peaches, then try including just a little spinach. Then add a little arugula. Add whatever nuts they like (almonds? pistachios?). If they'll let you, add a little goat cheese (or feta or blue cheese). Call it the "gradual gourmet" method.

Vinaigrette:

1½ cups fresh raspberries

1 batch Classic Vinaigrette (page 302; see Note)

Sea salt and ground black pepper, optional

Salad:

1 large or 2 small bunches baby spinach (about 12 ounces, or 1 large bag or clamshell)

4 large peaches, pitted and cut into bite-size pieces

½ cup sliced almonds, pistachios, or walnuts

1 cup loosely packed arugula

¼ cup crumbled feta, goat, or blue cheese, optional

1. Make the vinaigrette: Press ½ cup raspberries through a fine-mesh sieve set over a small bowl (discard the solids). Add the Classic Vinaigrette and whisk to combine. Taste and season with salt and pepper, if desired.

2. Make the salad: In a large salad bowl, gently toss 2 to 3 tablespoons of the prepared vinaigrette with the spinach, peaches, nuts, arugula, and cheese, if using (take care not to bruise the peaches). Reserve the rest of the vinaigrette to be added, as desired, on individual servings. (Kids often don't like salads that are overdressed—too "slimy"!) Garnish the salad with the remaining raspberries.

Note: If time is short (when isn't it?), use store-bought raspberry vinaigrette. Your kids will love it either way.

P E A R S

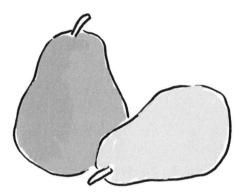

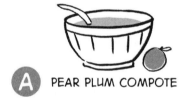

A PEAR PLUM COMPOTE

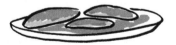
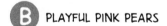

B PLAYFUL PINK PEARS

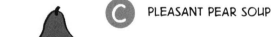
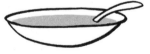

C PLEASANT PEAR SOUP

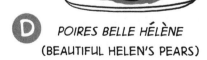

D *POIRES BELLE HÉLÈNE*
(BEAUTIFUL HELEN'S PEARS)

Pear Plum Compote

8 minutes to prepare (3 minutes hands-on); makes 6 to 8 baby jars

ON ITS OWN, PEAR COMPOTE CAN BE SLIGHTLY GRAINY, DEPENDING ON THE variety and ripeness of the pears. Combining pear with plum makes this compote smoother and just slightly more tangy—a nice contrast to the puréed apples and bananas your baby may already love.

> 1 ripe pear, peeled, quartered, and cored
> 1 large or 2 small ripe plums, peeled and quartered
> ⅛ teaspoon ground cinnamon

1. In a saucepan over high heat, bring 2 cups of water to a boil and then add the pears and plums. Reduce the heat to medium-high and simmer until very tender, about 5 minutes. Remove the pan from the heat and strain the fruit, reserving the cooking liquid.
2. In a blender, combine the cooked fruit, cinnamon, and ½ cup of the cooking liquid and purée until smooth. If needed, add more cooking liquid to reach desired consistency.

 Playful Pink Pears

25 minutes to prepare (5 minutes hands-on); serves 4 adults or older children

THE FLAVOR OF PEARS REALLY EMERGES WHEN THEY'RE TEAMED WITH SOMEthing slightly acidic. In this recipe, the cranberry juice does the trick. Plus it turns the pears bright pink, which creates a funny yet familiar dessert that will get your kids thinking about flavors.

> 3 cups cranberry juice (see Note)
> Liquid honey or stevia, to taste
> 2 whole star anise
> One 2- to 3-inch cinnamon stick or 1 teaspoon ground cinnamon
> 2 whole cloves
> 4 ripe pears, quartered and cored

1. In a medium saucepan over high heat, bring the juice, honey, star anise, cinnamon, and cloves to a boil, stirring well. Reduce the heat to medium-low and simmer for about 10 minutes, stirring occasionally. Add the pears in a single layer, cover, and simmer for about 5 minutes. Gently turn the pears over, and simmer for 5 more minutes, or until just tender. Remove the pan from the heat, leaving the pears in the syrup and the lid firmly on the pan to prevent the syrup from becoming too thick. (The heat will gradually cook the pears, but they'll stay firm.) Set aside until cool, then transfer the pan to the fridge to chill the pears completely. Serve the pears cold with the syrup.

Note: If desired, you can use cranberry cocktail instead of cranberry juice; just omit the honey or stevia.

Taste-Training Tip: As you're eating, ask your children to guess how the pears turned pink. For older children, you can have them compare the flavor with cranberry juice, cranberry sauce, or (best of all) frozen raw cranberries. Can they taste the cranberry flavor in the pears?

 Pleasant Pear Soup

15 minutes to prepare; serves 4 adults or older children

FOR YEARS, I AVOIDED FENNEL IN THE GROCERY STORE. *WHAT, EXACTLY,* I wondered, *am I supposed to do with it?* I just assumed my kids wouldn't eat it. As with so many foods, I was delighted to be proven wrong—it's now a Le Billon family favorite. The fennel has a slight anise or licorice taste to it, which makes this soup sweet but interesting.

    1 tablespoon salted butter
    2 tablespoons olive oil
    2 large or 3 small fennel bulbs, fronds removed, halved, cored, and cut into chunks
    1 medium onion, thinly sliced
    1 teaspoon sea salt
    ½ teaspoon ground black pepper

4 medium pears, peeled, quartered, and cored

2 potatoes, peeled and diced

1 cup apple juice

4 cups *Brodo* (page 301) or ready-to-use low-sodium vegetable broth

1 bay leaf

1. In a large saucepan over medium-high heat, melt the butter in the oil. Add the fennel, onion, salt, and pepper. Reduce the heat to medium, cover, and cook, stirring often, until the onion begins to turn golden brown, 5 to 6 minutes. Add the pears and potatoes, increase the heat to high, and bring to a rolling boil; cook for 2 to 3 minutes. Reduce the heat to medium, add the apple juice, *brodo*, and bay leaf, cover, and simmer, stirring often, until the fennel, pears, and potatoes are tender, about 5 minutes. Remove the pan from the heat and discard the bay leaf.
2. Using a blender, purée the soup until smooth. Serve immediately.

Adventurous Eaters Tip: Garnish with toasted fennel seeds for a crunchy, flavorful option.

Poires Belle Hélène (Beautiful Helen's Pears)

45 minutes to prepare (30 minutes hands-on); serves 4 adults or older children

THIS AMAZING DESSERT IS SLIGHTLY OUT OF FASHION IN FRANCE. IT WAS invented in the 19th century and named after an opera about Helen of Troy by Jacques Offenbach. My husband ate it a lot growing up, when it was one of the most popular desserts at dinner parties. Other desserts are more popular among the French these days—including, ironically, American crisps and crumbles, to which entire cookbooks are devoted—so it took me a few years in France before I discovered this dish. When I did, I was immediately hooked.

The poached pears are drizzled with chocolate syrup (and, in some recipes, crystallized violets). Simpler versions (like this one) use sliced almonds instead of the violets. The combination of sweet pear with dark chocolate is irresistible. Plus, it feels incredibly indulgent while still being pretty healthy. American or British versions often add cream-based sauces, but this version is faithful to the French original, which is deceptively simple. *Bon appétit!*

4 ripe pears, peeled, stems left on (see Notes)

1 tablespoon salted butter

4 ounces bittersweet or semi-sweet chocolate, chopped

½ cup half-and-half (10%) cream, whole milk, or milk alternative

1 teaspoon pure vanilla extract

¼ cup pure maple syrup

½ cup flaked or slivered almonds, optional (see Notes)

1. Make the poached pears: Using a paring knife, slice a thin layer off the bottom of each pear so that it can sit upright. Arrange the pears (upright) in a large saucepan and add enough water just to cover them. Remove the pears and set aside. Bring the water to a boil over high heat, gently lower each pear into the pan, and poach until the pears are tender when pierced with the point of a sharp knife, 10 to 12 minutes. (Don't undercook the pears: the goal is to have very tender pears that you can easily eat with a dessert spoon.) Using tongs, gently transfer the pears to a baking dish, discarding the poaching liquid. Cover and refrigerate to cool completely.

2. Make the chocolate sauce: In a small saucepan over low heat, melt the butter. Add the chocolate and cream and cook, stirring constantly, until the chocolate has completely melted. (Add a little extra cream if the mixture seems too thick—it should be pourable.) Remove the pan from the heat and set aside to cool slightly. (If the sauce becomes too thick, you can thin it by stirring in 1 teaspoon of water at a time.)

3. When the pears are cooled, core them using an apple corer or paring knife, working from the bottom to remove the seeds and leaving the stem intact. Set each cored pear upright in its own serving dish, drizzle with maple syrup, then with the chocolate sauce, adding enough so that each pear floats in its own little chocolate lake. Garnish with almonds, if using, and serve.

Notes: For this recipe, choose a variety of pear that holds up well when heated, such as Bosc pears.

For an added touch, toast the almonds in a dry skillet over low heat, stirring often, for 4 to 5 minutes or until just beginning to turn golden brown.

Taste-Training Tip: Once you have served this dessert once, experiment by adding new spices to the chocolate sauce. Ground cinnamon and ginger are popular options, or try orange zest. This is a great way to get your kids trying new flavor combinations. Why not let them take turns picking flavors and seeing how they turn out? Some families eat this with the maple syrup and nuts only—if you aren't chocolate fans, give it a try.

My younger daughter loved the first few bites—it was amazing that she ate any of it, as she always claims to not like pears. My husband and I loved the pears—even with just the maple syrup and nuts.   —BABETTE

I finally got my 9-year-old to eat fruit for dessert!   —FRANÇOISE

Great recipe, especially as we are trying to transition from having a sweet dessert every night to having fruit instead.   —MIRA

STRAWBERRIES

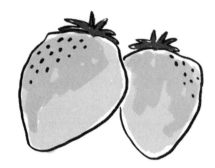

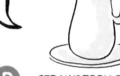
BERRY NICE!

B STRAWBERRY RHUBARB
SAUCE

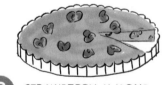

C STRAWBERRY ALMOND
CLAFOUTIS

D STRAWBERRY SPINACH
SALAD

Strawberry Rhubarb Sauce

15 minutes to prepare (5 minutes hands-on); serves 4 adults or children

THIS IS AN EXCITING, FUN PURÉE THAT DOUBLES AS A GREAT SAUCE FOR pouring over pancakes or splashing over ice cream. Or trickling over pound cake. Or spooning over morning oatmeal. Or drizzling over yogurt. Did I mention I like this sauce?

This sauce freezes well, so I make a large batch in early summer, when the strawberries and rhubarb are both ripe. In fact, I love this recipe so much that I started growing strawberries and rhubarb in our garden just so I can make it.

½ cup granulated sugar
2 cups chopped rhubarb stalks
2 cups hulled and sliced strawberries
1 ripe banana

1. In a medium saucepan over medium heat, bring ½ cup of water to a boil. Add the sugar and rhubarb and simmer until the rhubarb just starts to become tender, 3 to 4 minutes. Add the strawberries and simmer, stirring occasionally, until tender, 5 to 7 minutes. Add the banana and, using an immersion blender, purée the mixture, adding 1 teaspoon of water at a time to reach desired consistency. (Alternatively, transfer to a stand blender and purée.) Serve warm or cold, on just about anything!

Strawberry Almond Clafoutis

1 hour to prepare (15 minutes hands-on); serves 6 to 8 adults or children

CLAFOUTIS ARE THE FRENCH ANSWER TO STRAWBERRY SHORTCAKE: UNPREtentious and reliably delicious. The fluffy custard is easy to make. The almonds are mouth-wateringly good served with strawberries. What are you waiting for?

¼ cup salted butter
½ cup all-purpose flour
½ cup slivered or whole blanched almonds

½ cup granulated sugar, plus 2 teaspoons for garnish, optional

1 tablespoon cornstarch

Pinch sea salt

3 large eggs

¾ cup whole milk

1½ pints strawberries, rinsed, hulled, and quartered, plus a few more for garnish

½ cup slivered almonds, optional

¼ cup whipping (35%) cream, optional

1. Preheat the oven to 350°F. Grease a baking dish.

2. In a saucepan over low heat, melt the butter. Remove the pan from the heat and set aside.

3. In a food processor, combine the flour and almonds and pulse until the almonds are finely ground. Add the sugar, cornstarch, and salt, and pulse to combine. Add the eggs, one by one, pulsing after each to combine. Add the melted butter and milk and process just until the mixture forms a batter the consistency of heavy cream.

4. Spread the strawberries in a single layer in the prepared baking dish. Pour the batter gently overtop, taking care not to disturb the strawberries. Bake in the oven until puffy and set, about 40 minutes. Remove the pan from the oven and set aside to cool. Serve warm or cold straight from the dish. Garnish with a sprinkling of sugar or slivered almonds, top with fresh strawberries, drizzle with cream, or enjoy it plain.

Ⓓ Strawberry Spinach Salad

5 minutes to prepare (5 minutes hands-on); serves 4 adults or children

FOR MANY KIDS, THE SECRET TO ACCEPTING NEW VEGETABLES (EVEN THE typically disliked ones) is combining them with a bit of sweetness and healthy fat. (The good new is that healthy fat help us absorb nutrients, and the vitamin C in the strawberries helps us absorb the iron in the spinach.) Boiled spinach is no fun, but this salad is delicious. *Parfait!*

3 tablespoons extra virgin olive oil

1 tablespoon balsamic vinegar

1 teaspoon pure maple syrup

Pinch sea salt and ground black pepper

1 large or 2 small bunches baby spinach (about 12 ounces, or 1 large bag or clamshell)

1 pint strawberries, rinsed, hulled, and cut into bite-size pieces

½ cup slivered almonds, toasted

½ cup red onion, finely sliced, optional

1. In a large salad bowl, whisk together the oil, vinegar, maple syrup, salt, and pepper. Add the spinach, strawberries, almonds, and onion, if using, and gently toss to combine. Serve immediately (or else the spinach will wilt). *Voilà!*

Taste-Training Tip: If you're not sure your kids will like this, go back a step. Introduce them to the taste of spinach using some of the recipes on pages 221–225. Or toss some strawberries with the vinaigrette one day, just to try. They'll get there.

WATERMELON

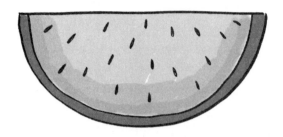

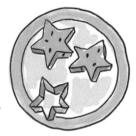

MELON LOVERS OF THE WORLD UNITE!

 WATERMELON STARS

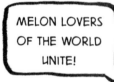 WATERMELON SOUP

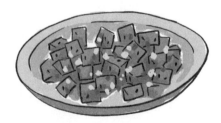 WATERMELON, LIME, AND FETA SALAD

Watermelon Stars

5 minutes to prepare (5 minutes hands-on); serves as many as you like

THIS SIMPLE, FUN RECIPE IS A GREAT WAY TO INTRODUCE TODDLERS TO watermelon. They'll love helping you make the stars. (Warning: this usually gets messy!)

1 small seedless watermelon

1. Cut the watermelon into slices about ¼ inch thick. Lay the slices flat on a cutting board or baking sheet. Using a cookie cutter(s), cut fun shapes from the watermelon (roundish shapes work best). (The leftovers make great juice—just blend, strain, and serve with a squeeze of lime juice. It will keep in the fridge for a day or two.)

Watermelon Soup

3 hours 10 minutes to prepare (10 minutes hands-on); serves 4 to 6 adults or older children

MAYBE IT'S BECAUSE I HAVE TWO LITTLE GIRLS, BUT I FIND PINK FOODS super-appealing. This soup can be served as a summer soup all on its own or as a dessert soup any time of year.

4 cups coarsely chopped watermelon (about ½ small seedless watermelon)
1 cucumber, peeled, seeded, and coarsely chopped
1 cup plain Greek yogurt, plus extra for garnish
Juice from 2 lemons or 4 limes (about 4 tablespoons)
Pinch sea salt
¼ cup chopped fresh mint leaves, for garnish
Liquid honey, for garnish

1. In a blender, combine the watermelon, cucumber, yogurt, lemon juice, and salt and purée until smooth. Transfer to an airtight container and chill for 3 hours (or overnight). To serve, ladle into bowls and garnish with mint and drizzles of yogurt and honey, if desired. (You may need to mix a bit of water into the yogurt for it to drizzle.)

Ⓓ Watermelon, Lime, and Feta Salad

7 minutes to prepare (7 minutes hands-on); serves 4 to 6 adults or children

MOST CHILDREN LOVE WATERMELON, SO THIS IS A GREAT WAY TO INTRODUCE them to feta cheese (which many young children adore, surprisingly). The three flavors of watermelon, lime, and feta remind me of southern France, where this is a traditional late-summer salad.

> 4 cups chopped watermelon (about ½ small seedless watermelon; see Note)
> 1 cup crumbled feta cheese
> ½ cup minced fresh cilantro leaves or minced fresh mint and basil leaves
> 10 black olives, pitted and chopped into small pieces, optional
> Juice of 2 limes (about 2 tablespoons) or to taste

1. Arrange the watermelon in a single layer on a serving plate and sprinkle with feta, cilantro, and olives, if using. (Do not toss!) Drizzle the lime juice over the entire plate, then allow guests to serve themselves.

Note: Watermelon cuts easily with cookie cutters. Use them to create a whimsical version of this salad for your child (have them help cut out the shapes).

Spice Is Nice: Desserts

(B)
(C)
(D)
Baby's Birthday Yogurt Cake with Chocolate Avocado Icing

1 hour 5 minutes to prepare (20 minutes hands-on); serves 8 adults or children (small slices)

THIS (RELATIVELY) HEALTHY YOGURT CAKE IS ONE OF THE MOST TRADI-tional French desserts and is often one of the first desserts that French children make at home. It's easy to make (and relatively hard to ruin). We love to serve this as a birthday cake—it's *that* good.

Yogurt cake has a simple, moist texture that children love. In fact, it's a lot like a pound cake, except without the butter (yogurt and vegetable oil are used instead). The lemon zest and slightly tangy flavor from the yogurt offset the sweetness of the cake nicely. Perfect at any time of day.

I've added a very North American twist: avocado icing. (Not well known in France, I must say!) It was a hit with my test families and is a lovely, creamy alternative to butter.

The cake can be made in advance and stored, tightly covered, in the refrigerator for up to 2 days, but the icing is best made right before serving.

Yogurt Cake:

1 cup plain Greek yogurt

¾ cup granulated sugar

2 large eggs

⅓ cup vegetable oil

1 teaspoon pure vanilla extract

1 tablespoon finely grated lemon zest

1⅔ cups all-purpose flour

1½ teaspoons baking powder

½ teaspoon baking soda

¼ teaspoon sea salt

Chocolate Avocado Icing:

2 large avocados, pitted and peeled

1 teaspoon pure vanilla extract

2 tablespoons unsalted butter, softened, optional

1 to 2 cups confectioners' (icing) sugar

¼ teaspoon ground cinnamon

¼ teaspoon sea salt

6 tablespoons cocoa powder

1. Preheat the oven to 350°F. Butter a 10-inch round cake pan and line the bottom with parchment paper.

2. In a large mixing bowl, whisk together the yogurt and sugar. Add the eggs one at a time, beating well after each addition. Add the vegetable oil, vanilla, and lemon zest and whisk to combine.

3. In a separate bowl, whisk together the flour, baking powder, baking soda, and salt. Fold the dry ingredients into the wet ingredients until just combined. (Don't overmix.)

4. Pour the batter into the prepared cake pan and bake in the oven until golden brown on top or until a knife inserted into the middle of the cake comes out clean, about 30 to 35 minutes. Remove the pan from the oven and allow the cake to cool in the pan for 10 minutes, then turn out onto a wire rack to cool completely before icing.

5. Make the icing: In a food processor, combine the avocado, vanilla, and butter, if using, and process until smooth. With the motor running, add 1 cup sugar a little bit at a time, followed by the cinnamon, salt, and cocoa powder. Add up to another 1 cup sugar, to taste. If the icing is a little chunky, try gradually adding a little bit of cream until you achieve the desired consistency.

6. Ice the cake: Transfer the cake to a serving platter. Using a spatula, place a large amount of icing on top of the cake, in the center. Gently smooth out the icing toward the edges until the top is evenly covered. Cover the sides with icing. Smooth the sides by slowly spinning the plate while holding the spatula to the icing surface. Repeat with the remaining icing until the top and sides are evenly covered.

Taste-Training Tip: If you're really adventurous, frost your cake with gorgeously green Lemon-Avocado Icing instead. Follow the directions above, substituting 1 tablespoon lemon juice for the cocoa powder and adding at least an extra ½ cup confectioners' sugar to achieve the right consistency. For this version, serve the cake immediately after frosting—it tends to turn brown with time.

I made the Chocolate Avocado Icing for my son's birthday. There were 10 kids present and not one of them blinked an eye at it. It looks—and tastes—exactly like regular chocolate icing!
—Roberta

The cake even by itself is delicious: it's fairly dense and the lemon flavor is lovely. With the icing, it's amazing.
—Teresa

Almond Mini-Cakes (*Financiers*)

35 minutes to prepare (10 minutes hands-on); makes about 2 dozen

THESE LITTLE ALMOND TEA CAKES ARE UTTERLY IRRESISTIBLE. IN THEIR small, rectangular version, they are often served as an after-dinner *mignardise* (the name comes from the old-fashioned French word *mignard*, meaning a small child, particularly a graceful, sweet one). Sums them up perfectly!

Wonderful bonus: these are gluten-free, as they use almond flour instead of wheat flour. If you can't find almond flour, you can make your own by using your food processor to grind up blanched almonds. The consistency won't be as fine, but the cakes will still be yummy!

6 tablespoons salted butter
1 cup almond flour

¾ cup confectioners' (icing) sugar

4 tablespoons cocoa powder

⅛ teaspoon sea salt

2 large egg whites

¼ teaspoon pure almond extract

1. Preheat the oven to 375°F. Lightly grease a mini-muffin pan.

2. In a small saucepan over low heat, melt the butter. Remove the pan from the heat and set it aside to cool (if the butter is too hot, it will cook the egg whites—disastrous!).

3. In a large mixing bowl, whisk together the flour, sugar, cocoa powder, and salt. Stir in the egg whites and almond extract, then gradually stir in the cooled melted butter and mix until smooth.

4. Pour the batter into the mini-muffin pan, filling each cup about three-quarters full. Bake in the oven until the cakes are puffy and slightly springy to the touch, 12 to 15 minutes. Remove from the oven and set aside to cool completely (if you try to remove them from the molds while they're still warm they'll break!). The cakes will keep for up to a week stored in an airtight container at room temperature.

Adventurous Eaters Tip: Substitute ½ teaspoon crumbled culinary lavender for the almond extract.

No-Bake Choco-Raisin Treats (*Mendiants*)

60 minutes to prepare (30 minutes hands-on); makes about 8 large cookies (1 ounce each) or 16 smaller cookies (½ ounce each)

THESE FUN CHOCOLATE TREATS TASTE DECADENT BUT ARE (RELATIVELY) low in sugar—and they're a lighter alternative to filling chocolate cake. Who would have thought something this easy to make could be so delicious?

A *mendiant* (the traditional French word for this dessert) is a chocolate disk studded with nuts and dried fruits: raisins, hazelnuts, figs, and almonds. Traditionally eaten at Christmas, they're now eaten year-round, and endless varieties can be found that incorporate everything from seeds to fruit peel. Use your imagination! The goal is to have your children enjoying making food and being in the kitchen, so try to make these together.

1 tablespoon unsalted butter

8 ounces dark or milk chocolate, chopped

1 teaspoon ground cinnamon

1 tablespoon whipping (35%) cream (if you are using dark chocolate)

½ cup slivered or sliced almonds

½ cup dried blueberries

1. In a small saucepan over low heat, melt the butter. Add the chocolate and stir constantly, until completely melted. Add the cinnamon and, if using dark chocolate, the cream.

2. Assemble the cookies: You can do this using either silicone muffin cups (my preference) or parchment paper. If using muffin cups, drop about 1 heaping tablespoon melted chocolate mixture into the bottom of three or four muffin cups at a time. If using parchment paper, lay the parchment on a flat work surface and drop small spoonfuls of chocolate on the sheet, about three or four at a time, using the back of the spoon to make little circles about 2 inches in diameter. Before the chocolate hardens, add the almonds and blueberries in any design you like—use your imagination! (If the chocolate mixture hardens before you have finished, don't worry: you can remelt it.)

3. Set the cookies aside to harden, testing the edges cautiously until you are sure they are ready (at least 30 minutes). *Yum!*

Taste-Training Tip: I've suggested blueberries and almonds in this recipe, but start with toppings your children already love, then introduce new flavors. Toppings can include nuts (almonds, pistachios, praline, pecans), dried fruit (raisins, blueberries, thinly sliced apricots, cranberries, crystallized ginger or orange rind), or even fleur de sel, seeds, or chunks of your favorite cookies.

My 4½-year-old loved making these with me. She did all the stirring and added the fruit and nuts. We made them 5 days ago, and she's still asking for the chocolate cookies each night after dinner! —BABETTE

These were a hit with my boys (ages 6 and 4). They declared them the best cookies that I've ever made and had fun adding granola and fresh raspberries and strawberries as toppings. —STACY

Cinnamon and Clove Biscuits

10 minutes to prepare; makes 2 dozen small biscuits

TEETHING BABIES LOVE TO GNAW ON ALMOST ANYTHING, BUT TRADITIONAL baby biscuits are fairly plain. Why not spice it up? Clove oil is traditionally used to help soothe toothaches, and this recipe uses a bit of ground clove to give the biscuits a unique taste.

1 cup dry infant oat cereal

1 cup all-purpose flour, wheat flour, or oat flour

1 teaspoon ground cinnamon

½ teaspoon ground cloves

6 tablespoons melted butter

1 cup very ripe banana, mashed until smooth (about 2 bananas)

1. Preheat the oven to 425°F. Line a baking sheet with parchment paper.
2. In a large mixing bowl, whisk together the cereal, flour, cinnamon and cloves. Gradually stir in the butter, then mix in the banana. (The dough should be soft and smooth; if it is too dry, add 1 tablespoon of water at a time—how much you'll need will depend on how large and ripe the banana is.)
3. Using your hands, form the dough into a ball and then roll it out on a floured work surface to ¼-inch thickness. Using a cookie cutter, cut into circles or ovals (no pointy edges or corners for baby!). Transfer the shapes to the prepared baking sheet and bake in the oven until lightly browned, 7 to 10 minutes. Remove from the oven and set aside to cool completely on the baking sheet before serving. The cookies will keep in an airtight container at room temperature for up to 1 week.

Safety Tip: As with any teething biscuit, watch your child closely to make sure the biscuit doesn't pose a choking hazard.

B

C

D

Lemon Mousse

2 hours 20 minutes to prepare (10 minutes hands-on); serves 4 adults or 8 children

WHEN YOU MENTION THE WORD "MOUSSE," MOST PEOPLE THINK OF CHOCOLATE. But lemon mousse is wonderful, too. With very little cream, this mousse is a light and airy, melt-in-your-mouth treat.

> 4 large eggs
> 1 cup granulated sugar
> ¼ teaspoon sea salt
> Zest of 2 lemons (about 1 heaping tablespoon)
> Juice of 2 lemons (about 4 tablespoons)
> ½ cup whipping (35%) cream
> ½ teaspoon pure vanilla extract
> Garnish: very thin lemon slices, fresh berries, or fresh mint leaves

1. Make the lemon curd: In two small bowls, separate the egg yolks from the whites, setting the whites aside for later.
2. In a chilled, medium saucepan, whisk together the egg yolks and ½ cup sugar, then whisk in the salt and lemon zest and juice until smooth. Cook the mixture over medium heat, stirring often, until thickened to the consistency of a not-quite-set pudding, about 10 minutes. Pour the mixture through a fine-mesh sieve into a large bowl (discard any solids). Cover with plastic wrap and chill in the fridge until firm (at least 1 hour, longer if possible).
3. Make the mousse: In a bowl, whisk together the egg whites and the remaining ½ cup sugar until stiff peaks form, then gently fold in the chilled lemon curd. In another bowl, whisk together the cream and vanilla until stiff peaks form. Fold the whipped cream into the lemon mixture until just combined (don't overstir).
4. Spoon the mousse into individual serving ramekins or little cups and chill for at least 1 hour, or until firm to the touch. Serve with your choice of garnish.

Safety Tip: This dish does include raw egg, which according to medical advice in some countries should not be given to babies under 12 months.

ⒷⒸⒹ Roast Pineapple Surprise

20 minutes to prepare (5 minutes hands-on); serves 4 adults or 8 children (depending on the size of your pineapple)

THIS SIMPLE YET DELICIOUS DESSERT IS REALLY QUICK. PREPARE THE PINE-apple as your dinner is cooking, then let it bake while you're eating. It's a classic French approach: lots of fruit, a little sugar, and an intriguing flavor twist.

> 1 ripe pineapple
> ¼ cup packed dark brown sugar
> ½ teaspoon ground ginger
> ½ teaspoon ground cinnamon
> ½ teaspoon ground allspice
> Juice of ½ lemon (about 1 tablespoon)
> Vanilla or coconut ice cream or gelato, for serving

1. Preheat the oven to 325°F. Line a baking sheet with parchment paper.
2. Remove the pineapple's spiky leaves by twisting them away from the crown. Core the pineapple. Using a sharp knife, cut the unpeeled pineapple into slices approximately 1 inch thick. Arrange the slices in a single layer on the prepared baking sheet.
3. In a small bowl, combine the brown sugar, ginger, cinnamon, allspice, lemon juice, and ¼ cup of water. Drizzle the mixture over the pineapple slices. Cover tightly with aluminium foil. Bake in the oven for about 15 minutes, or until tender, basting once or twice with the juice in the pan. Serve with ice cream. *Yum!*

ⒷⒸⒹ Lemon Ginger Thyme Shortbread

1 hour 30 minutes to prepare (15 minutes hands-on); makes at least 2 dozen cookies

SHORTBREAD IS A PERENNIAL KIDS' FAVORITE. THIS RECIPE SPICES IT UP with a bit of ginger and thyme. Sounds odd, I know, but trust me: this is a delicious combination.

3 cups all-purpose flour

¼ teaspoon sea salt

2 teaspoons baking powder

1 teaspoon dried thyme

1 cup unsalted butter, at room temperature

1 cup granulated sugar

2 tablespoons lemon zest

1 teaspoon ground ginger

1 large egg

Juice of 1 lemon (about 2 tablespoons)

¼ cup whole milk

1. Preheat the oven to 325°F. Line a baking sheet with parchment paper.

2. In a large bowl, combine the flour, salt, baking powder, and thyme. Set aside.

3. Using a stand mixer on medium-high speed, cream the butter, sugar, lemon zest, and ginger until fluffy, 3 to 5 minutes. Add the egg and lemon juice and mix on medium speed until combined. Add the flour mixture and mix on low speed just until incorporated (don't overmix). Divide the dough in half and, using your hands, shape each piece into a log (they'll be about 3 inches thick). Wrap in plastic wrap and chill in the fridge for at least 1 hour (or freeze for 15 minutes).

4. Unwrap the dough and cut the logs into ½-inch-thick slices. Arrange the cookies 1 inch apart on the prepared baking sheet. Using a pastry brush, brush the cookies with milk. Bake in the oven for 12 to 15 minutes, or until the edges turn golden. *Yum!*

Warm Chocolate Ginger Fondant Cake

1 hour 35 minutes to prepare (20 minutes hands-on); makes about 1 dozen small cakes

THIS DESSERT HAS A SOFT CENTER THAT OOZES OUT OF THE CAKE WHEN YOU cut it. That's why these are baked in little muffin cups or ramekins—so everyone can enjoy the ooze at their own pace. The most important step in this recipe is buttering the muffin cups really, really well so that the mini-cakes can slide out onto a plate without breaking.

⅔ cup salted butter

4 ounces dark chocolate, chopped into ½-inch pieces

⅔ cup granulated sugar

4 large eggs

½ cup all-purpose flour

1 teaspoon ground ginger

Vanilla ice cream, for serving, optional

1. Grease 6 muffin cups or ramekins, line with paper muffin liners, then butter the muffin liners (important!).
2. In a small saucepan over low heat, combine the butter and chocolate and gently stir until completely melted.
3. Meanwhile, in a large mixing bowl, combine the sugar and eggs and beat until the mixture is pale, thick, and just starting to stick together (pastry chefs refer to this as a "ribbony" texture, because when you lift your mixing spoon the batter pours back into the bowl in thick ribbons).
4. In a separate bowl, mix the flour and ginger until well combined. Stir the flour into the egg mixture until combined, then add the chocolate mixture, stirring until smooth. Pour the batter into the (well-greased) muffin cups, then cover with plastic wrap and chill for at least 30 minutes or, preferably, 1 hour. (If you're using ramekins, I suggest arranging them on a baking sheet before you pop them in the fridge.)
5. When you are nearly ready to serve, preheat the oven to 400°F. Bake until the top of each cake is set, 12 to 13 minutes. Remove from the oven and set aside for at least 5 minutes to cool. Serve warm, all by themselves, or with a little vanilla ice cream, if desired.

Taste-Training Tip: Experiment with this recipe to vary the flavor: try adding 1 teaspoon pure vanilla extract or ½ teaspoon pure almond, orange, or lavender extract. Or try adding 1 teaspoon ground cinnamon or substituting 1 teaspoon dried mint for the ground ginger. Make a game out of asking your kids to guess which flavor you've added.

B

C

D

Cat's Tongue Cookies (*Langues-de-Chat*)

17 minutes to prepare (10 minutes hands-on); makes at least 2 dozen cookies

THESE EASY-TO-MAKE COOKIES ARE LITERALLY MELT-IN-YOUR-MOUTH delicious. Experts will tell you to use a piping bag to get precise shapes, but for kids, I simply recommend that you let them spread the batter on their own to create lots of fun shapes.

½ cup unsalted butter

½ cup confectioners' (icing) sugar

3 large egg whites

½ teaspoon pure vanilla extract

1 cup all-purpose flour

¼ teaspoon sea salt

Zest of 1 lemon

1. Preheat the oven to 375°F. Line a baking sheet with parchment paper, then generously grease it with butter. (Trust me, do not put these cookies on the baking sheet directly, even if it is well greased: they will likely break when you try to remove them.)

2. In a stand mixer on high speed, cream the butter until smooth. Add the sugar and beat until fluffy. Beat in the egg whites, then add the vanilla and mix until incorporated. Using a wooden spoon, gently fold in the flour and salt, scraping down the sides of the bowl as needed, then stir in the lemon zest.

3. Using the back of a spoon, spread the batter onto the baking sheet in "cat's tongue" shapes (roughly oval), then bake in the oven until the cookies start to turn golden at the edges, 5 to 7 minutes. Remove the baking sheet from the oven and immediately slide the cookies onto a wire rack to cool (if you let them cool on the baking sheet, they'll be more likely to break when you remove them—do it while they're still warm). Cool completely before serving.

Taste-Training Tip: Try serving these cookies alongside other desserts, such as the Lemon Mousse (page 295) or *Verrines* (page 300) to add a little texture contrast.

Verrines (The No Fuss, No Muss, Elegant Dessert-in-a-Glass)

10 minutes to prepare (10 minutes hands-on); serves 6 to 12 (depending on the size and shape of your glasses)

Ⓑ
Ⓒ
Ⓓ

VERRINES ARE A STANDBY IN FRANCE, SERVED AS APERITIFS (WHEN YOU'D be likely to find layers of savory ingredients like avocado and crab mousse) or dessert. The way they are served says a lot about the French approach to food: it needs to be a feast for the eyes as well as for the stomach. Your *verrine* will look a lot like a parfait, and you'll serve it with a spoon. The kids will be intrigued by the layers and will soon be asking to make their own. I've suggested a basic recipe below, but the standard method is to alternate dairy and fruit layers. Be creative—the possibilities are endless.

Choose clear, narrow glasses for serving. A small juice glass might work well, or even a wine glass, but forgo the traditional sundae-size container—this is a "less is more" dessert.

> 1 recipe Pear Plum Compote (page 277)
> 1 cup plain Greek yogurt
> 1 cup fresh blueberries and raspberries, for garnish

1. In each glass, carefully spoon about 4 tablespoons pear plum compote. Using a clean spoon, carefully top each with about 4 tablespoons yogurt, creating a clean second layer. Repeat until you have the desired number of beautiful layers. Garnish with blueberries and raspberries. Serve immediately or refrigerate and serve within a few hours.

Friendly Flavors: Basic Recipes

Brodo (Vegetable Broth)

35 minutes to prepare (5 minutes hands-on); makes about 2 cups

Brodo is the Italian word for "broth," which is precisely the right way to describe this vegetable soup: subtle and tasty. Italian parents make this broth in batches and either freeze or refrigerate it. At first, they serve it on its own, but it quickly becomes the basis for other soups and purées. Italians are told by their pediatricians to mix this broth with rice cereal and to add a dollop of olive oil and a sprinkle of grated Parmesan (Parmigiano-Reggiano) before serving. This results in a melt-in-your-mouth *pappa* that Italian babies love.

1 medium potato, peeled and cut into 1-inch cubes
1 large carrot, peeled and chopped
1 large zucchini, chopped
1 small baby leek, white part only, thinly sliced, optional

1. In a large saucepan over medium heat, simmer the potato, carrot, zucchini, and leek in 4 cups of water until the liquid is reduced by half, about 30 minutes (as the mixture simmers, it will thicken). Strain the soup through a fine-mesh sieve (discard solids) and set aside to cool.

Note: This recipe can easily be doubled. *Brodo* will keep in the fridge (tightly covered) for 2 to 3 days and in the freezer for well for up to 1 month.

Friendly Flavor Tip: Use *brodo* as a base for your baby purées or soups. It will lend a rich underlying flavor that kids will find reassuringly familiar, which will help them get acquainted faster with new foods and tastes as you vary the purée/soup recipes.

~~~~~~~~~~~~~~~~~~~~~~~~~~~~~

(B)
(C)
(D)

Classic Vinaigrette
2 to 3 minutes to prepare (2 to 3 minutes hands-on); makes about 1 cup

THIS VINAIGRETTE IS INCREDIBLY VERSATILE. SERVE IT AS A SALAD DRESSING or as a dip for vegetables. Before the main evening meal, for example, I serve the vinaigrette in little individual bowls along with crudités (raw vegetables) such as carrots and cucumber sticks. For snack, sometimes my daughters prepare veggie trays in mini-muffin tins, filling each hole with different veggies and one hole with vinaigrette. Kids like cute things and fun presentation!

The vinaigrette will keep in an airtight container in the fridge for up to 1 week. It saves money and is healthier than store-bought, too.

½ cup extra virgin olive oil or other high-quality vegetable oil
¼ cup vinegar
½ tablespoon Dijon-style mustard
1 tablespoon pure maple syrup, optional
1 tablespoon finely minced shallot, scallion, or onion, optional

1. In a resealable glass jar, combine the oil, vinegar, mustard, maple syrup, and shallot and shake vigorously. Taste before serving and adjust the seasonings to your preference (my mother-in-law, for example, prefers a more acidic vinaigrette, whereas I prefer a slightly sweeter, gentler version).

Taste-Training Tip: Kids love using the vinaigrette as a dip (my younger daughter would eat it with a spoon if I let her!). Once they are familiar with this flavor, encourage your child to try new veggies by dipping them in the vinaigrette.

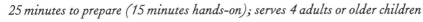

B

C

D

Quick Crunchy Casserole

25 minutes to prepare (15 minutes hands-on); serves 4 adults or older children

THIS CASSEROLE IS BASED ON THE FRENCH GRATIN COOKING TECHNIQUE, used to serve a variety of vegetables, from potatoes to cauliflower. *Gratin* refers to a white sauce and crunchy topping that lends savory flavor to vegetables. Once kids are used to gratin-style dishes, this is a wonderful way to get them to try new foods: the gratin sauce and topping provides a reassuringly familiar look and taste to accompany the new food.

This is a great dish to prepare in advance: store it in the fridge and pop it in the oven when you get home. Double the cooking time (at least) if you're putting this in the oven straight from the fridge.

> Vegetables, such as: 5 or 6 large carrots, peeled and cut into bite-size pieces; 5 large
> potatoes, peeled and thinly sliced; or 1 large or 2 small heads cauliflower, cut into
> florets
> 3 tablespoons salted butter, plus 2 tablespoons for topping
> 3 tablespoons all-purpose flour
> 2 cups milk
> ½ teaspoon ground black pepper
> ¼ teaspoon ground nutmeg
> 1 pinch sea salt, optional
> ¾ cup dried breadcrumbs
> ¾ cup grated Parmesan cheese

1. Preheat the oven to 400°F.
2. In a large saucepan over medium-high heat, bring 6 cups of water to a rolling boil. Add the vegetables and cook until crisp-tender, 5 to 7 minutes, depending on the veggie and its cut. (Do not overcook—you don't want mushy veggies.) Drain the vegetables and set aside.
3. Meanwhile, make the white sauce: In a medium saucepan over medium heat, melt 3 tablespoons butter. Increase the heat to high, add the flour, and cook, whisking vigorously, for 1 minute (make sure the mixture doesn't burn). Add the milk, reduce the heat to medium (not too low), and cook, stirring constantly, for 2 to 3 minutes, just until the sauce begins to thicken. Add the pepper, nutmeg, and salt, if using.

4. Pour the veggies into a baking dish and cover evenly with the sauce. Set aside.

5. In a small bowl, combine the breadcrumbs and Parmesan. Sprinkle the mixture evenly overtop the casserole. Dot with 2 tablespoons of butter cut into small pieces. Bake in the oven for 8 to 10 minutes, or until the topping is golden brown and crunchy.

Taste-Training Tip: When you first make this dish, use a vegetable your children already like. Once they like the gratin-style, start adding different vegetables. Ask your kids to think of combinations they'd like to try—the possibilities are endless.

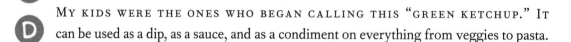

B C D *Pistou* (aka "Green Ketchup")

17 minutes to prepare (10 minutes hands-on); makes about 1 cup

MY KIDS WERE THE ONES WHO BEGAN CALLING THIS "GREEN KETCHUP." It can be used as a dip, as a sauce, and as a condiment on everything from veggies to pasta.

½ head broccoli, cut into florets (about 2 cups)
¼ cup fresh basil leaves
1 tablespoon extra virgin olive oil
3 teaspoons grated Parmesan cheese
1 tablespoon fresh lemon juice
⅛ teaspoon dried thyme or ¼ teaspoon fresh thyme leaves
½ cup roasted unsalted sunflower seeds, optional
½ cup *Brodo* (page 301) or ready-to-use low-sodium vegetable broth
Sea salt

1. Bring a medium saucepan of water to a boil over medium heat. Add the broccoli and cook until soft, 7 to 8 minutes. Strain the broccoli, reserving the cooking liquid.

2. In a food processor or blender, combine the cooked broccoli, basil, oil, Parmesan, lemon juice, thyme, sunflower seeds, if using, and ½ cup of the cooking liquid and purée until smooth. Add salt to taste (I personally don't salt my *pistou*, but some do). *Pistou* keeps well stored in an airtight container in the fridge for up to a week. I sometimes freeze what I don't use in little ice-cube trays (although this changes the texture slightly); it will keep for up to a month in the freezer.

Acknowledgments

Getting to Yum was a labor of love to which many people contributed.

For tolerating my sometimes weird, sometimes wonderful attempts in the kitchen, my warmest thanks to two dozen test families scattered around the world: Babette, Benoite, Beth, Brandy, Celine, Claire, Elena, Françoise, Greg, Hélène, Jacqueline, Jamie, Jennifer, Jessica, Jon, Joy, Kristine, Lori, Roberta, Virginie, Martha, Meg, Mira, Sarah Jane, Shaylagh, Sophie, Stacy, Teresa, and Trevor, and their families, and all the children and caregivers at the Alphabet Academy—the most dedicated taste testers I could ever have hoped for.

Martha Magor Webb wore many hats: agent, taste tester, supportive critic, and friend. It's been a joy to work with her. Thanks, too, to the entire team at the Anne McDermid Agency.

Designing and daydreaming about illustrations with artist Sarah Jane Wright was the perfect inspiration for writing. Thanks, Sarah Jane, for your willingness to brainstorm and your endless patience.

Thanks, too, to Judy Phillips, proofreader extraordinaire.

Kate Cassaday (HarperCollins Canada) and Cassie Jones (William Morrow in New York) were, once again, a delight to work with: savvy, creative, insightful, and kind. I'm grateful to them and their colleagues for the enthusiasm they showed from beginning to end.

Last but not least: to Sophie, Claire, and Philippe—for your patience and for your loving, honest criticism. Who else would have put up with some of my wackier kitchen experiments? If I ever doubted that "food is love," you've put those doubts happily to rest.

Index

treats
 vs. food, 95–96
 homemade, 96
 in moderation, 12, 51
 outside the home, 166
tree nuts, 177
trigger foods, 124
turmeric, 194
turnip, 144
tweens, 165
Twitter, 43

umami, 34
 games about, 34–35
under-nutrition, 90
United Kingdom, 60
urination, 156

variety
 for babies, 139–41, 142, 150
 in France, 98
 games about, 7, 100–106
 health benefits of, 49
 psychological benefits of, 96
 rotation rule for, 96, 106, 153, 163
 seasonal foods for, 99, 107
 during taste testing, 30
 techniques for increasing, 97–98
 for toddlers, 163
 "try something new every day" rule for, 97, 106
vegetables
 for babies, 143–45, 146–47
 child-led, 110
 cooking for babies, 151
 defined, 112
 flavor ladder for, 178–79
 food illiteracy about, 42
 genetic modification of, 90
 health benefits of, 67
 during pregnancy, 142
 raw, 97
 sweet, 90

top 10, 178–79
 veggies or fruits first ritual, 76–79, 80, 95, 156
 washing, 97
vending machines, 44
Verrines (The No Fuss, No Muss, Elegant Dessert-in-a-Glass), 300
Vicious Carrots, 190–91
Vij's, 197
vinaigrette, 302
viral marketing, 43
Virginie (parent), 47
vision, and appetite, 123
vitamin C, 147, 225, 284
vitamin deficiency, 11
vitamin pills, 49
vocabulary, 53

walnuts, 177
Wansink, Brian, 45, 83, 123, 124, 125
Warm Chocolate Ginger Fondant Cake, 297–98
Warm Spinach Citrus Salad, 224–25
wasabi, 20
water, 72, 96
watercress, 143
watermelon, 286–88
Watermelon, Lime, and Feta Salad, 288
Watermelon Soup, 287
Watermelon Stars, 287
weaning
 from juice, 66
 from kids' food, 93–96, 106–7
 from processed food, 91
websites, marketing on, 43
weight control, 128
West, Mae, 189
whale meat, 18
wheat, delaying for babies, 177
White-Out Campaign, 148
white sauce, 196
winter squash, 143

women
 comfort foods of, 125
 as supertasters, 22
words, about food, 30

yogurt
 Baby's Birthday Yogurt Cake, 289–91
 food illiteracy about, 41
 Perfect Blueberry Parfait, 259–60
 Tangy Citrus Smoothie, 267–86
 Verrines (The No Fuss, No Muss, Elegant Dessert-in-a-Glass), 300
Yogurt Game, 105–6
yogurt tubes, 94
Yummy Yellow Purée, 194

Zesty Orange Salad, 269–70
zinc deficiency, 11
zucchini, 238–42
 as a first food, 143
 Melt-in-Your-Mouth Zucchini Purée, 239
 Quick Zucchini-Ham Quiche, 241–42
 Roasted Zucchini with Cumin, 239–40
 Sophie's Spinach Surprise, 221–22
 Zucchini Flan, 240–41
Zucchini Flan, 240–41

ALSO BY KAREN LE BILLON

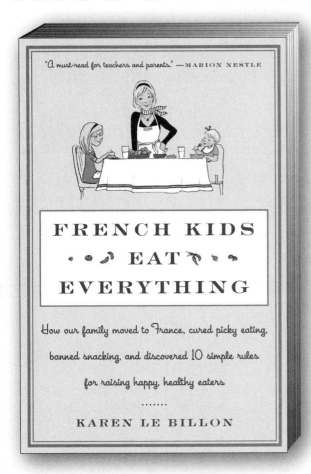

FRENCH KIDS EAT EVERYTHING
How Our Family Moved to France, Cured Picky Eating, Banned Snacking, and Discovered 10 Simple Rules for Raising Happy, Healthy Eaters

Available in Paperback and eBook

French Kids Eat Everything is a wonderfully wry account of how Karen Le Billon was able to alter her children's deep-rooted, decidedly unhealthy North American eating habits while they were all living in France. At once a memoir, a cookbook, a how-to handbook, and a delightful exploration of how the French manage to feed children without endless battles and struggles with pickiness, it features recipes, practical tips, and ten easy-to-follow rules for raising happy and healthy young eaters.

"A breezy but practical volume for hurried parents looking to keep their kids well-fed. . . ."
—*Publishers Weekly*

"A must–read for teachers and parents."
—Marion Nestle, Professor of Nutrition, Food Studies, and Public Health at New York University and author of *What to Eat*

"A book that every parent of young children will want to read. . . . Humorous as well as instructive, this culinary adventure will change the lives of parents and children alike."
—Patricia Wells, author of *The Provence Cookbook*

"A fascinating and valuable read." —Lynne Rossetto Kasper